MULTIPLE SCLEROSIS

HUMAN HORIZONS SERIES

MULTIPLE SCLEROSIS:
A PERSONAL EXPLORATION

by

ALEXANDER BURNFIELD

A CONDOR BOOK
SOUVENIR PRESS (E & A) LTD

First published 1985 by Souvenir Press
(Educational & Academic) Ltd,
43 Great Russell Street, London WC1B 3PA

Reprinted 1986 (twice), 1987, 1988, 1991, 1996, 1998

ISBN 0 285 65019 X casebound
ISBN 0 285 65018 1 paperback

Printed and bound in Great Britain by
The Guernsey Press Co Ltd, Guernsey, C.I.

This book is dedicated to Gilbert Macdonald who was Chairman of the Multiple Sclerosis Society of Great Britain and Northern Ireland from 1976 until his death in 1983. The pages that follow owe much to his friendship and, like many other people who have multiple sclerosis, I shall always be grateful to 'Mac' for his inspiration and encouragement.

Foreword

by Shelagh Macdonald
wife of the late Gilbert Macdonald, and a tireless worker with him on behalf of people with multiple sclerosis

I did not know much about Dr Alexander Burnfield when I first set eyes on him. He was a young doctor, his friends called him Sandy, and he had multiple sclerosis.

He was a distant figure on a platform in Edinburgh. I was late for the MS meeting, and heard only the last few minutes of his talk – and that I did not hear well, lurking unobtrusively as I was at the very back. But I did hear the audience's response, and felt the stimulated atmosphere in the hall.

The next time I heard Sandy talk I turned up on time. This was a London meeting of people with MS and those involved in their lives.

I have heard a lot of talks on multiple sclerosis – some excellent, some good, some boring, some irritatingly superior and some downright unhelpful. But this one was different, and I sensed that everyone in the room felt the same.

The first most noticeable thing was that Sandy, without apparent conscious effort, spoke to the meeting as if he were talking to each person individually. He might have been in one's own living-room, chatting over a coffee, making the odd joke, telling an occasional human tale.

But it wasn't only his manner that was refreshing. He also talked about MS in a way that I believe few there had encountered before – except, maybe, from especially perceptive friends or relations. There was nothing mealy-mouthed about him. He talked honestly yet gently, un-shirkingly yet understandingly. He knew the problems from the inside – but had the objectivity of a good doctor. (He can be objective about doctors, too!)

On the faces there I could see all kinds of things: relief, pleasure, concentrated interest, often laughter. Just about everybody had a question to ask. They felt they could ask him anything - as they'd ask a friend. And they did. Then, when answering questions, he did not glance away from difficulties or gloss over painful matters, or treat people's anxieties as trivial.

It all comes across in this book. You will feel he is talking to you, not telling you things. He covers pretty well every aspect of MS that anyone involved or interested could wish to know about - in such a way that he is sharing his observations and feelings, not informing you that he knows best.

He is especially helpful on the tricky areas that so many people, doctors included, find so difficult to deal with: anger, grief, disbelief, self-pity, resentment and guilt - in marriages, families and society. He talks sensibly and openly about sex and pregnancy. He is also very helpful on the practicalities - what to expect from the illness and why, different effects on different people, professional help, treatments, allowances, diets, fads and fancies, exercise and fun, work, everyday problems. Throughout, he relates what he says to human experience - his own and his wife's and the many people with MS whom he has met and talked to.

Most of all, he compassionately conveys his understanding of the dark struggle from the time of diagnosis to the point of reaching some acceptance - yet not giving in. He talks out of knowledge, because he has 'been there', but also, I believe, because of an unusual insight into others.

Not everyone, unfortunately, can have Sandy sitting chatting in the living-room - he does quite enough as it is. But now you have this book, and it's a pretty good replacement.

London, 1985

Contents

Acknowledgements

Special thanks are due to my wife, Penny, for the help that she has given me in writing this book, and for her enduring patience and support. Josephine Burnfield, my sister-in-law, did most of the typing and Rosemary Davis took over after the birth of Josephine's baby. I would like to express my gratitude and admiration to them both for their hard work and useful comments.

I am grateful to the following people for their valuable and constructive suggestions, as well as for their time and expertise: Carolyn Evans, Wendy Goodall, Dr Philip Kennedy, Professor Lindsay McLellan, John Walford, OBE, and Shirley Winch. Thanks also go to the many friends who have given me inspiration and encouragement, particularly Tony Banks, Cynthia Benz, Kathy Llewelyn, Terry Lister and my father-in-law, Frank Fuller.

I am much indebted to all those associated with the Multiple Sclerosis Society of Great Britain and Northern Ireland for the parts they have played in the creation of this book, especially Nadia Bocock, Margaret Bown and Rita Saupin, and also to Beverley Brown and Deanna Groetzinger of the Canadian MS Society, together with Joanna McLean of the MS Society of Western Australia. Catherine Dobson, Meriel Gwyther and Sue Henshaw of the Education Centre Library at the Royal Hampshire County Hospital, Winchester, have provided me with an efficient back-up service, and to them I express my sincere appreciation.

There is a special place in my heart for those people whose experiences I have used in this book. To maintain confidentiality identities have sometimes been disguised by altering names and obscuring details. I respect them for their courage and remember them with gratitude. Finally, I should like to thank Sophie Owen for taking the photographs and Tessa Harrow of Souvenir Press for her help and encouragement.

A Personal Introduction

Exhausted after playing tennis for only a short time, I bent down, picked up the ball to serve, and had an unpleasant shock. The top half of Uncle Bunt was missing in a blurred haze! Even now, as I think back to that moment, I can still see his long baggy trousers and large brown shoes. Although I did not know it then, this was my first meeting with multiple sclerosis, known as MS for short.

I served the ball regardless and, a moment later, it reappeared from nowhere to hit me on the face. This was too much and, making some excuse about the sun in my eyes, I abandoned the game. I went indoors to sit in the cool and to regain my composure. I experimented with my vision, squinting at various objects, covering each eye in turn. It was not long before I realised that a large area of vision was missing when I used my left eye on its own. The upper half of anything I looked at with that eye was not there. If I looked at a face I just saw the mouth and chin. When I examined a clock I could only see the numbers from four to nine. Looking at a cluster of red roses only with my left eye, I noticed that they appeared pink and that there were not so many of them. The right eye was working normally, revealing the full cluster of bright red roses.

All this happened twenty years ago when I was in my second year at medical school and on a weekend visit home. It had been a hot afternoon in June and my sixty-year-old uncle and I had been playing at the farm where my family lived and where I had been brought up. I remember feeling ashamed that I had to give up the game with my strong and healthy farmer uncle, and ashamed that he, who was forty years older, had more stamina than I.

By the time that I saw the doctor responsible for student health at my medical school, I had developed further symptoms. There was an aching pain behind my left eye, and this became sharp and knife-like if I moved the eye from side to side. The doctor examined my eye, but to my surprise he insisted on examining every other part of me as well. He spent much time with my knee jerk and he seemed to fiddle for ages with a key that he ran along the outside of the soles of my feet. Until this time I had naïvely assumed that the whole trouble was in my eye. I had received little training in clinical medicine at that stage, but this doctor's neurological examination alarmed me – he seemed to have a grave look on his face. I pumped him with questions which he answered briefly and evasively.

This was the start of many more examinations and investigations; I went on to see an ophthalmologist, then a technician who plotted my visual fields, and after another visit to the Eye Department, I ended up seeing a neurologist. My anxiety increased but questions and conversation were discouraged. 'Optic neuritis' was given as the cause of my symptoms, and I was assured that it would probably clear completely. The cause? 'There are lots of possible reasons' – but I noticed that my neurologist averted his eyes and changed the subject.

I went off to the library at the medical school and took out some textbooks on ophthalmology and neurology. I discovered that there were indeed several possible causes for my condition, most of them quite rare. But the commonest cause was multiple sclerosis: I read that the majority of people who presented with optic neuritis developed MS within about ten years or so, although some would have no further neurological symptoms.

I was numbed with shock; I sat frozen to my seat in the library, feeling apart from those around me, who now seemed unreal. I was alone and frightened. Sweat dripped off my face, and I felt my heart beating fast and loud in my head. Would I develop MS? No, I would be one of the lucky ones. But I could not believe that, either.

At the next appointment I asked the neurologist whether he thought that I might have MS. Looking away quickly, he said that if I could read the textbooks I knew as much as any doctor, and that only time would tell. This was not reassuring - the textbooks in the library had painted a gloomy picture of MS. A person with this disease could become paralysed within ten to twenty years, and might end up blind, unable to speak, or incapable of controlling his bladder and bowels. Premature senility could occur and death usually resulted from chest or urinary infection or from massive bedsores. It all seemed unreal and couldn't happen to me - or could it? I did not feel able to question the neurologist about these things. It would have seemed 'bad form'. Still less could I express my emotional feelings, my fears, sadness and anger. I did not want to upset him. So I kept my thoughts to myself, and felt more alone than ever.

Over the next few weeks the pain in my eye lessened and then disappeared. My vision also improved but I was left with a 'blind area' in the upper part of my left visual field. The neurologist saw me for a final appointment and wrote a letter about me to the student health doctor. Like so many others in a similar position, I found an opportunity to open the letter and read its contents - I desperately wanted to know the truth. My neurologist was one step ahead of me in this particular game. The letter did not mention the dreaded words 'multiple sclerosis' at all; instead it said, 'He has had an attack of optic neuritis in his left eye and is aware of the possible future implications.'

Neither of my doctors offered me a follow-up appointment; it was assumed that I would return only if further symptoms occurred. But I did not return. I continued to do my work as a medical student over the next three years. I was continually aware of the 'blind spot' and could never forget that other symptoms might develop at any time. I could not talk to other people about my fears, whether family or friends, and as a result there were times when I felt isolated and different from other people. A part of me refused to accept the possibility of MS, and yet another part of me would never let it go.

Penny, my medical student girlfriend, knew that I had had an attack of optic neuritis, and she also knew that MS could develop. Despite this, she was prepared to accept me as I was, and bravely she said that she would take a chance on the future. Still students, we married one year before my final examinations, and two years before hers. Unlike many couples, we married knowing that MS could occur and having discussed the possibilities. Because of this, I think that our personal problems have been less than they might otherwise have been.

I qualified as a doctor in May, 1968. But before being allowed to practise my craft on an unsuspecting world, I had to complete a pre-registration year. This was divided into two halves: six months of surgery and six months of medicine. My first appointment was as House Surgeon to the Neurosurgical Unit. This was a demanding and prestigious post, which required that I gain a deep and practical knowledge of neurology and neuro-anatomy. I was to be plunged fully into the world of brain surgery and of the neurologist. It is not difficult to imagine how mixed my feelings were; apprehension and curiosity wrestled with one another in my mind.

I found that there was to be no escape from MS. My duties included covering for the House Physician to the Neurology Department on alternate evenings and weekends. I was therefore regularly in contact with and sometimes responsible for the management of those patients who had MS. These unfortunate people were often severely disabled and fitted almost exactly the frightening descriptions that I had read in the text-books as a student. Some of my work was in the operating theatre assisting the neurosurgeons, but I avoided this when I could. It involved standing still for long periods, something that I could not do. I was sometimes reprimanded for leaning heavily, moving unsteadily, and being restless. To tell them that I might have MS seemed silly, and I did not think that I would be believed. Besides, I wanted to prove that I was healthy and normal.

Although tired and occasionally depressed, and often without much sleep, I managed to present an acceptable front and to behave in the 'jokey' and superficial way that seems to be expected of people working in the knife-edge world of life and death. I learned much from this job for which I am grateful. How difficult it is, as a doctor, to tell the truth, to face the bereaved, and to make decisions about people's lives – especially when all I wanted was to sleep. At the end of this job I was able to drill holes in skulls, to co-ordinate medical services for a road accident victim at 3 am in the morning, and to support nurses caring for a child dying from a brain tumour. I had been thrown in at the deep end, and my own worries about MS seemed of little importance. Who was I to think of my own health, when in the morning I had to tell a young couple that their four-year-old daughter was brain-damaged after an accident, and that it was doubtful whether she would live? The temptation was to spend as little time as possible with people, so as to avoid the pain of sharing grief and shock. I began to see my own neurologist in a different light!

Once Penny had qualified, we moved to Winchester and I began work as a Casualty Officer. I had been working for only six weeks when I noticed that my right hand was numb. Within two days I had lost the use of my right arm which had become clumsy and awkward. The nurses in Casualty took over the notes for me since my writing had become illegible. I could not suture cuts and wounds and I asked the nurses to help with these and with other surgical procedures. We all knew that there was something wrong, but no one was going to admit it. I felt a fool and was particularly conscious that some people were trying to pretend that nothing unusual had happened. Was I being treated differently? Were people avoiding me? I felt a freak, but I was eventually persuaded by a colleague to see another neurologist.

Dr Graveson told me bluntly that I did have multiple sclerosis and that I should have come to see him earlier. The definite diagnosis was a relief and I was grateful for this man's frank approach. I felt a burden drop away, but a part of me still did not want to believe that I really had MS. In a subsequent meeting with my new neurologist I was given the chance to talk about my future. He said that the outlook was uncertain, but I could expect progressive disability and my plans should make allowance for this. He wondered whether I had considered entering a speciality like radiology or some branches of pathology which would be less demanding. I could think of nothing worse; I had always hoped to train as a psychiatrist after gaining more medical experience.

After some months, and with encouragement from senior colleagues, I began my new psychiatric training. The next few years were not easy and, because my MS did not show outwardly, I tried to continue to present a normal image to others as an able-bodied person. I felt guilty about having the disease, and ashamed of mentioning it to other people. My family seemed to prefer to minimise or to deny it as much as possible – just like me. Over the next few years I had several more MS relapses. Optic neuritis occurred in my right eye and returned in my left eye, making my vision even worse. I had episodes of vertigo, accompanied by nystagmus (rapid flicking of the eyes from side to side), and when I was very tired I noticed a dull pain in both eyes, numbness in my right hand, and a heavy feeling in my left leg.

Towards the end of my psychiatric training, and about three years after the diagnosis was confirmed, I underwent a personal analysis. This was in order to help me understand and accept myself better, so that I could increase my skills as a psychotherapist. This experience enabled me to work through the unhealthy guilt associated with my MS (was I ill because I was bad?) and I came to understand much better the religious conditioning that had influenced my emotional growth and personality development. I was able to make contact with parts of myself that I had hidden or had feared, and to accept myself more fully as a separate and worthwhile individual. My analyst, Dr Lotte Rosenberg, died only sixteen months after we started this work together. She remains an inspiration to me and I shall always be grateful to her for freeing me from self-doubt, guilt, fear, and many prejudices. She also helped me to live with love and self-acceptance. Her death, combined with the worsening of my MS, brought on a severe depression. In desperation I raided the hospital pharmacy and gave myself a course of antidepressants – at that stage I did not seem able to share my troubles with anyone else. Penny was busy working as a trainee in General Practice, and she too found my MS depressing. We were both in the same boat, and it was not easy to help one another. The antidepressants did help a little, but it was counselling from a colleague that finally broke the spell and enabled me to come to terms. Maria was having problems with her marriage and children and she was also depressed. We were able to relate to each other as equals and as ordinary human beings, not as the two psychiatrists that we both were. Neither of us was superior or inferior to the other. We shared our concerns and listened to one another with care and respect.

Maria accepted my anxieties and my sad, angry and confused feelings. She helped me to understand that these feelings were natural and realistic. I realised from talking to her that I would have been abnormal not to have been emotionally upset by a very real loss of health and threat to my security. I was able to express my feelings openly after this, to admit to having MS, and to make realistic decisions about my future. For the first time I felt that I had been understood; I had received counselling from another person, who happened to be a doctor.

Once I had made the decision to allow for my MS, and once I had accepted the disease as a real part of me whether I liked it or not, I joined the MS Society. My own depression had left me and was replaced by a desire to help other people who had the same difficulties in accepting the disease or who had other emotional and relationship problems associated with MS. I also wanted to explain what I had learned to other doctors, many of whom seemed to be ignorant of the psychological side of multiple sclerosis. At the same time, I wanted to help myself by doing something positive about my own disease: to turn base metal into gold.

This book is the record of my personal exploration into the world of MS and reflects what I have seen, heard and discovered on my 'travels'. It has been an adventure with all the dangers, hardships and surprises that characterise any journey into uncharted territory. Yet I have also found purpose, understanding, and other treasures when I have looked for them. It is my hope that what I have discovered will help others who, like me, are destined to spend time in this mysterious and often terrifying world, and that this book will also help to make multiple sclerosis clearer to those people, whether volunteers or professionals, who attempt to understand and to help us.

Update 1996

It is now over ten years since this book first came out, and a lot has happened, both in the MS world and to me and my family. As in previous reprints, I have updated bits and pieces here and there, mostly when dealing with research, treatment and organisational changes. The main part of the book, dealing with the personal effects of MS, remains as before.

I am not as young as I was – fifty-one and a grandad! I still walk with a stick, but I no longer have my pedal tricycle: this has been replaced by a three-wheeled electric scooter. I keep fit, still work for the NHS and now chair the International Federation of MS Societies' *International Conference Committee*.

Penny is well, and so are Clare and Sarah, their baby daughters and our old Collie, Jemma. Finally, THANK YOU to all those people living with MS in the family who have sent so many interesting and encouraging letters – it has made writing this book a pleasure in spite of all the horrors of MS.

Sandy Burnfield

1 · The Disease

I had just ordered a headstone for my father's grave and, accompanied by my mother, we were leaving the stone-mason's yard. The mason himself had been particularly helpful, and was seeing us off the premises. Just as we were saying good-bye to him and thanking him for his help, he motioned to me to stay for a while. In a conspiratorial voice he enquired, 'I see that you have a limp and walk with a stick; could you tell me what your particular trouble is?' I saw nothing wrong in his interest, and told him that I had multiple sclerosis. He looked thoughtful, and then said, 'Oh, I am sorry to hear that. Is it something that is likely to take you soon?'

I was left rather speechless at this question, which is unusual, as anyone who knows me will confirm. I was taken aback at his directness and the implication that MS might lead to my death. I hope that I covered up my momentary confusion at what I regarded as a somewhat tactless thing to say, especially coming from a stonemason. In the few seconds of silence between his question and my answer, many visions and thoughts went through my mind, including how much custom he was expecting to get out of our family! Eventually I replied, 'MS in my case has lasted for nearly twenty years, and I am relatively little disabled. I hope to live a long time yet.' Nevertheless, the whole experience had certainly shaken me. I do not normally think in terms of death, certainly as far as my MS is concerned, but his possibly innocent question made me think again.

The Image of MS
MS definitely has a bad press. When you first mention the subject to people they will often think the worst. Some will be embarrassed and will not know what to say next. Others are extremely sympathetic and almost overwhelming in their sorrow for your future. MS has sinister significance to people because usually they know only of the worst cases in the community, and only the worst cases are being actively treated by GPs or hospital doctors. This negative and serious image of MS is only part of the truth.

There is no doubt that a few people with the disease have a rapidly progressive course and over a short period of time, maybe less than five years, they will become seriously disabled, and may even die. But these are a minority and it is important to realise that most people with MS live normal lives and may never need to use a wheelchair. Many with the disease will have a long life span and will be only a little disabled, even in old age.

MS – The First Description
So what exactly is MS? When was it first discovered? what causes it, and how does it affect those who suffer from it?

I am not a neurologist or a pathologist. I am someone who has lived with MS for a long time; I am also a qualified doctor. and I work as a psychiatrist. For this reason I shall not be giving detailed medical information about MS, but I shall look at the disease in a way that I hope will be helpful to many people with MS, their friends and relatives who have to live with a disease often mysterious in its complexity.

MS has been recognised as a disease for only just over one hundred years. In 1868 the French neurologist, Charcot, first made the connection between symptoms experienced by some of his patients and a certain type of damage to the brain and spinal cord of these patients found after death. Charcot's patients were seriously affected by the disease and the signs of illness that he first observed included 'intention tremor', 'scanning speech' and a medical condition called 'nystagmus'.

In ordinary English, an 'intention tremor' means that someone has difficulty in controlling their movements when they try to carry out a specific action. A neurologist will often ask a patient to try to touch his or her nose; people with an intention tremor find that, as their hand gets nearer to their nose, it will wobble increasingly and move about in a clumsy manner. The same action is needed in order to drink a cup of tea or to strike a match, and indeed, someone with an intention tremor can be quite badly disabled.

The second of Charcot's symptoms, 'scanning speech', can be a feature of MS when a person is badly disabled. The speech is affected so that the person talks in a jerky manner, rather like a Dalek. This is because the co-ordination of the tongue and other muscles is impaired in the same way that there is a loss of control in the arms or legs when someone has an intention tremor.

Charcot's third symptom, 'nystagmus', is a rapidly fluctuating movement of the eyes, often present when a person looks from one side to another.

These three abnormalities of muscle control are sometimes seen when damage has occurred in a part of the brain which deals with fine co-ordination. Charcot discovered that they were related to 'sclerotic plaques' or scars localised in certain areas of the central nervous system, and he described the disease as 'sclerose en plaques'. In English it was known as disseminated sclerosis, and this name lasted for many years until, by international agreement, it was standardised to multiple sclerosis. Many people are under the impression that disseminated sclerosis is a different condition from multiple sclerosis, but this is not so.

The Cause of Symptoms

The 'scars' in the brain and spinal cord that Charcot discovered were the reason for the symptoms that occurred in his patients, and similar scars are the cause of all the various symptoms that occur in MS. The scars, or sclerotic plaques, develop following inflammation around certain nerve fibres, and they are associated with the loss of the 'myelin sheath'. The myelin sheath surrounding each nerve fibre is like a layer of insulation, and when it is lost nerve impulses are slowed down or cannot go along the fibre at all (Fig 1).

If the nerves do not work, or work badly, messages do not arrive from sensory areas in the skin, eyes, or from other parts of the body such as joints. This causes symptoms such as numbness, loss of position sense or visual difficulties. Or if the nerves are those that carry messages from the brain to the muscles, then weakness or clumsiness might occur. This can lead to symptoms of MS such as difficulty in walking, weakness in the arms, problems in moving the eyes together (causing double vision) or lack of co-ordination of the tongue. Sometimes inflammation with consequent scarring occurs in a part of the brain responsible for the general co-ordination of the nervous system, called the 'cerebellum'. When this happens the person will experience problems with balance and control over movements, and there may also be a tremor.

When plaques of sclerosis occur in the brain or spinal cord it is possible that symptoms will develop; but this is not inevitable. Sometimes a person will experience very few symptoms; yet when they die (for one reason or another) a lot of demyelination and sclerosis can be found which has apparently led to the production of hardly any symptoms. On the other hand, sometimes a few scars situated in important areas of the brain or spinal cord can cause serious disability.

The characteristic pattern of MS is damage due to demyelination occurring in *separate places* in the central nervous system and produced at *different times*, and this is the basis of the clinical diagnosis of the disease. (See Chapter 4.)

Who Gets MS and Why?
Why do some people get MS and others not? This is an interesting question and, although we know some of the answers, the picture is not yet clear. In Britain, MS affects

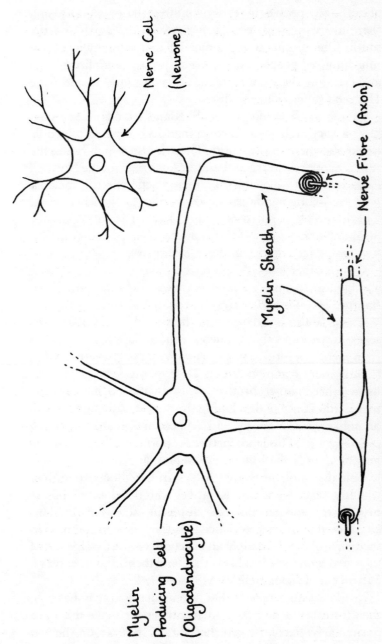

Fig 1. Myelin sheath wrapped around nerve fibres (not to scale).

about sixty people in every hundred-thousand, although there are variations, especially between the north and the south. One recent survey indicated that as many as one in nine hundred people have either suspected or confirmed MS and certainly there are more than fifty thousand people in the UK who suffer from the disease.

People in the Orkney and Shetland Islands of Scotland have a very high risk of developing MS compared to people living elsewhere in the world. There is also a high risk in the rest of Scotland, in Ireland and in some parts of the North of England. This is possibly due to a genetic effect, associated with the Viking invasions, but this cannot be the whole story. The high risk is not present in all countries of Viking or Scandinavian origin; for instance, people living in the Faeroes or Iceland do not have a high risk.

On the other hand, MS is uncommon among the Chinese and Japanese and completely absent among pure bred Bantus, Eskimos and native American Indians.

There is also a difference in the way that MS affects the sexes, for we know that women are more likely to develop MS than men, in a ratio of three to two. We also know that MS is slightly more common among close relatives. Someone who has a father, mother, brother, or sister with MS, has a slightly increased chance of developing the disease, although it is still an unlikely event. People with MS commonly share the same 'tissue group'. This lends further support to the importance of genetics, and I shall mention it again later.

This does not mean that MS is an hereditary condition, which it certainly is not. Relatives who develop the disease may share some particular predisposing factor for MS. This might be due to an experience that they have in common in their environment (possibly an infection) or due to some sort of inherited tendency. It is likely that both these influences play a part in the development of MS (see Fig 2).

It is interesting to note that, if one identical twin has MS, then the other, who has an identical genetic make-up, is not particularly likely to get the disease. But he or she has

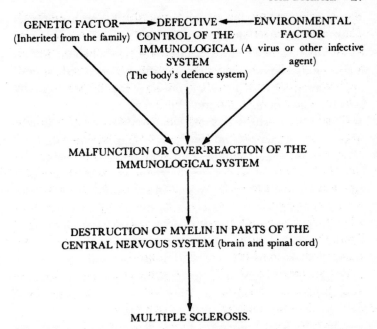

Fig 2. A possible sequence of events leading to MS.

a greater risk than an ordinary brother or sister of an affected person. This makes it clear that the genetic factor is only part of the story and that another part may be influences shared by families living in the same environment.

An American study of the early life of identical twins, one of whom has MS, found that the twin with the disease had more frequent infections in childhood than the one without MS. One study on its own cannot be taken as final, since it needs to be confirmed by others, but this is yet more evidence that an environmental factor plays a part in the development of MS.

I know two identical twin sisters one of whom, Julie, has MS. Julie and Janet are both married now and live in different places, but when they were children they were, naturally, brought up together. Julie had a mysterious fever when she was about three-and-a-half years old and, in the next few years of her life, she had more trouble with infectious diseases than her identical twin sister. It is tempting to speculate that the fever experienced by Julie when she was an infant may have been the reason for her subsequent development of MS. Janet did not have the fever or so many infections in her infancy and childhood.

It should be stressed that, whatever the environmental factor may be, there is no evidence to suggest that MS, once acquired, is an infectious or contagious disease. People can be assured that they cannot catch MS from someone who has it. In other words, MS is not spread in the same way as a cold, 'flu or chickenpox.

The most common age for MS to occur is around thirty years of age. It is less likely to occur in ages going away from thirty in either direction. So it has been found that a large proportion of people first developing MS are between the ages of twenty and forty, although there are still a few who develop the disease at a younger or older age.

What, then, is the cause of MS? It must be said straight away that, at the moment, nobody really knows. There are, of course, many theories and there are also the results of many years of research which give us some ideas about possible factors that could play a part in the development of MS. The first of these is the evidence gleaned from population studies. MS occurs much more commonly in certain areas and in certain populations than in others. As I have said, people in the northern European countries, in particular, have a high risk of developing the disease compared with people elsewhere. This increased risk also applies to people in countries where the majority of the population have come from northern Europe, such as Canada, New Zealand and Australia.

The incidence of MS is much higher in England than South Africa. Studies have shown that, if someone emigrates from England to South Africa before she is fifteen years old, she is less likely to develop MS than if she had stayed in England. On the other hand, if someone emigrates *after* the age of fifteen, she carries the increased risk of developing MS, as though she had stayed in England. This study is further evidence that there is an environmental factor in MS as well as a genetic factor. In other words, something must happen to people before they are fifteen years old which decides whether or not they will have a higher risk of developing the disease. More studies of this sort are being carried out on immigrants to other countries where it is possible to obtain a large enough sample. One of these is Great Britain, where there has been a significant number of immigrants from many different countries of the Commonwealth over several generations.

Research has looked into the genetic aspects of MS. I have already discussed the fact that MS is slightly commoner in close relatives than it is among people who are unrelated. It has been found that we all have 'tissue groups' in the same way that we all have blood groups. The interesting thing is that people who have MS are more likely to share certain tissue groups than people who do not have MS. It is thought that these tissue groups are related to one of the genetic factors in MS and that they may be associated with the body's defence mechanisms against infections known as the 'immunological system'.

All this is scientific fact, but I would like to speculate a little further. Apparently people who have MS are less likely to suffer from hepatitis, most cancers and leukaemia. Research into the genetic aspects of MS has suggested a possible reason for this. Long ago, when the people on this earth were very primitive, the genetic factor which now predisposes to MS could have had a useful function. It might have prevented overwhelming infections occurring, like hepatitis or septicaemia, which were major causes of death in Stone Age man who rarely lived more than twenty-five years.

If this is true, does it mean that my ancestors survived, because of their special genetic make-up, to live their full twenty-five years? But in my own case, living in the twentieth century, this same genetic factor no longer serves a useful function since I am unlikely to die from the same diseases as my Stone Age ancestors. It is actually causing me problems because I have lived much longer than my twenty-five years!

In MS it certainly seems that the body's defence mechanism is not working normally. There is some evidence that a particular group of white blood cells, (lymphocytes) responsible for controlling the immunological response, are not functioning properly, or are fewer than they should be. When the body's defence system is called into action in order to attack some particular invading organism, such as a virus, perhaps it does not stop when it should and goes on to cause damage to the nervous system.

Infection

An infective agent is thought to be one of the likely causes for the environmental influence that I have already mentioned, and various viruses have been suspected. In particular the measles virus, herpes virus and canine distemper viruses have all been suggested as possibilities. Another idea put forward is that the 'scrapie agent' may play a part in the development of MS. Scrapie is a virus-like organism that affects sheep. Interestingly, some vets researching a similar disease of sheep, swayback, developed MS several years later. But the cause of the swayback proved to be copper deficiency.

Current opinion, however tends towards the view that MS is associated with an as yet unidentified delayed-action virus acquired in childhood. Another possibility is that the disease agent is a 'germ' completely unlike a normal virus or bacteria. Agents of this sort are known to be responsible for the rare Kuru and Jakob-Creutzfeld diseases, both of which are characterised by progressive neurological symptoms and loss of intellectual function.

Sometimes reports are made claiming that certain viruses have been identified in the microscopic examination of tissues from people with MS. These reports have not been consistently repeated, and at the moment there is *no* firm evidence that one particular virus plays a part in MS. It could be that people with MS are susceptible to more than one type of virus or even to a combination of viruses. Because genetic factors may cause a defect in the immune defence system, viruses may either remain in the body for longer than they should, or the attempt to rid the body of them may cause damage to the nerve tissues. This latter effect is called an 'auto-immune reaction', and it is a characteristic of other diseases apart from MS.

Current Research

MS is a very complicated condition and research is taking place on a broad front. Some scientists are studying the effects of viruses on brain tissues; others are examining different populations to discover what it is that people with MS have in common, what is different about them from other people who do not have the disease.

Other research workers are trying to improve the methods of making a diagnosis and, recently, good progress has been made in this area. We now have the Magnetic Resonance Imager (MRI Scanner) which can safely and easily show up quite small patches of demyelination in the brains of people who have MS.

Some scientists are testing out new drugs or treatments under controlled conditions. One such drug is Beta Interferon. Experiments have convinced the authorities that it could be an effective treatment for some types of MS, and the manufacturers have now been given a licence enabling doctors to prescribe it in some well defined situations (see pp. 54–5). The value of polyunsaturated fatty acids like sunflower seed oil is still being assessed in this way, and possible anti-viral and immune-suppressant drugs are being researched. The controversy about Hyperbaric Oxygen treatment is being properly looked at under strictly scientific conditions to see whether in fact it does have a part to play. Proper scientific research of this sort is essential if we are to get a true picture of what possible treaments can really do, rather than relying on prejudice, wishful thinking, or on someone's financial greed!

A particularly important area of research is that of immunology, for this is now considered to be one of the keys to the cause of MS. MS Societies finance much of the research that is taking place into the disease and details of the research projects receiving grants are available from them. The Societies also publish journals and newsletters giving details of research findings written in lay language, together with sensible advice for people who have MS.

MS can affect different people in so many different ways that it is sometimes very hard to believe that it is a single condition. In fact some people think MS could be a collection of different diseases which all result in a similar sort of damage to the nervous system but for which there are different causes. One thing that points in this direction is evidence that if someone develops 'optic neuritis' (which is characterised by blurred vision and pain in an eye) as a first symptom of MS, and if this takes place in the spring or summer, the long-term outcome will be better than if the same symptom first developed in the winter or autumn. This is only an early finding, and more research is needed into this aspect, but it does seem to indicate that in these two instances a different sort of infective or allergic agent may be playing a part.

The diagram on page 27 shows the various factors that can play a part in the development of MS.

I like to compare the factors that may lead to MS with a fruit machine. A person will only 'win the jackpot' (develop the disease) if a certain pattern of fruits occurs when the machine is used, such as three oranges in a row. In MS one orange might represent a genetic factor, another orange might represent an infective agent and the third orange might represent another unknown factor, probably something to do with the immunological system. If you have a genetic pre-disposition but not the other two factors you will not develop MS and, in the same way, if you have an infective agent like a virus but do not have the other two factors, you will still not develop MS. But if you are unlucky enough to have all three oranges then MS will occur – a negative jackpot!

2 Symptoms

MS is a complicated disease and no two people will appear to have exactly the same symptoms. There are very many ways that the illness can affect people, and I can think of a number of friends of mine with MS who have completely different problems. James is a man in his middle age who has experienced gradually increasing weakness in both legs associated also with difficulties with his bladder now resulting in incontinence. He has never had a spell without symptoms and his condition has just got progressively worse and worse. James now has to use a wheelchair and he has aids to help his incontinence.

On the other hand, Susan developed MS when she was twenty-five years old, after her first child. She became rapidly disabled and was admitted to hospital paralysed. The situation at the time seemed very bleak. However, Susan recovered from this incident and has been able to walk again and to continue to live at home and bring up her child. Since that time she has remained relatively free from symptoms which have tended to come and go, but which have never resulted in long-term disability.

Jill's major problem is fatigue. She always looks perfectly normal and no one could ever guess that she has had MS for about twenty-five years. Her vision is occasionally blurred and she has had problems with her ability to touch and feel things with her hands and feet. This has sometimes led to numbness and to a burning pain in her legs, and to other odd feelings which come and go. However, Jill's main symptom of fatigue is only evident when she is very tired or hot and on these occasions she becomes more obviously disabled, almost a different person.

George also has MS. He looks physically fit and extremely active but he does not drive a car. This is because his vision in both eyes has been seriously affected and he is now registered as partially sighted. He uses special aids to help him see things, and even with these he has great difficulty in reading. Despite this, George has had few other symptoms, although he does get fatigue after exercising and he has, on physical examination by a doctor, signs of MS which are not visible to other people outside the consulting room.

There is one other person with MS whom I should like to mention. This is a young man called Julian. Julian has only had the disease for three years and he can walk with a stick, although in a very wobbly manner. He and his wife have two children but Julian no longer works and has lost an extremely interesting and well-paid job. This is because his main disability is his loss of concentration and memory. He finds it hard to work out simple problems, or to remember things, and his wife has become increasingly frustrated and depressed, despite the fact that Julian is relatively cheerful.

When I think of all these different people with MS, and when I remember others with different sorts of difficulties and problems, I then contrast them with myself. My MS appears, so far, to have been relatively benign and I can get about and do most things with little trouble. It is this immense variability in the course of the disease which leads some researchers to speculate that the term 'MS' may cover a collection of diseases, each of which results in a different pattern of damage to the nervous system.

Relapses and Remissions

One of the main characteristics of MS is the relapsing and remitting course it often follows. This means that episodes of disability (called relapses) occur which are followed by a recovery period known as a remission. Someone might have one MS symptom and then go five years or more before another symptom occurs. The period in between these two relapses could be completely uneventful. In the early stages,

MS usually starts with a single symptom like tripping over small obstacles, double vision, or perhaps blurred vision with pain in the eye. It is impossible to make a diagnosis of MS at this time for good reasons, since there are many other different causes of symptoms like these. If further incidents occur, separated by months or years, then these can be diagnostic of MS, with symptoms spaced out in time and related to different parts of the brain and spinal cord.

But although this is the usual pattern in MS, and the majority of people will experience the relapsing and remitting picture, a proportion of people become gradually disabled with no remissions. Earlier I mentioned James who has this progressive sort of MS. In his case, MS came on at an older age than usual, and he has not had any remissions at all. His MS has mainly affected his legs and bladder and he has sexual difficulties due to a variable type of impotence.

As I mentioned in the previous chapter, some unlucky people have a short and extremely severe form of MS, and studies have shown that about five per cent of people who contract the disease will be dead within five years. On the other hand, a number of people who develop MS will have practically no disability at all, even in old age, and this group is described as having a 'benign form' of the disease. People with benign MS frequently have sensory symptoms, rather than weakness, and the disease often starts with an attack of 'optic neuritis'. Most people probably fall between these two extremes and are disabled at some stage of their lives, increasingly so as time passes. But even they will not need to use a wheelchair all the time, and only a small proportion of people will end up severely disabled, bedridden or permanently confined to a wheelchair.

Quite often people ask whether MS will cause death. This is certainly one of the anxieties people have when they are first diagnosed, and it can also be a worry for relatives. The fact is that very few people indeed die from MS, which is a disabling disease, not a killing one. If people become severely disabled and their physical condition deteriorates, there is a possibility that they might die from one of the complications of MS, such as a respiratory or a urinary infection, but they are unlikely to die from the neurological damage itself. In fact many people who have MS die from something completely different. Like everyone else, as they get older they are likely to contract a more life-threatening condition than their MS, like heart disease or cancer.

Common Symptoms

The symptoms of MS are variable, but certain ones are more common than others. Optic neuritis, which is caused by demyelination in one or both of the optic nerves, usually results in blurred vision affecting areas of the visual field, and can result in blind spots known as 'scotomata'. In my own case, I have developed a patch of blurred vision in each eye, but with both eyes open my vision is relatively good.

A friend of mine, Helen, has described her own symptoms in a particularly clear way.

> I experienced a severe pain in my right eye, which lasted for several months. The pain developed quite suddenly and was of an aching nature, rather reminiscent of the ache one experiences after a tooth has been extracted. It was accompanied by an unpleasant sensation of a cold wind blowing into my eye. The area above my eye, near the bridge of my nose, was quite tender. This pain has recurred periodically and I have noticed, since its onset, the development of blurred, foggy patches in my vision in that eye.

Another common early symptom is 'diplopia', which is the medical word for double vision. Double vision can occur very early in MS and (like optic neuritis) people may remember having had this problem many years before they developed other signs of MS. Another common symptom is clumsiness of one arm, due to demyelination in the spinal cord blocking the messages coming from the joints and other parts of the arm.

Sensory Symptoms and Pain

Pins and needles, or numbness in the hands and feet, can be early symptoms of MS, and some people also have a strange tingling, or painful sensations in their legs, arms or trunk. Helen has described her symptoms as follows:

> For nearly eight years I have had numbness in my arms and legs whenever I lie down. More recently, in addition to this, I felt stabbing pains in my fingers and toes, sometimes enough to make my hands cold and clammy.

A few people experience a particularly unpleasant pain in the face, of a shooting and stabbing nature. This is known as trigeminal neuralgia because it affects the trigeminal (fifth cranial) nerve of the brain which carries the sensations of touch from the face area. The pain of trigeminal neuralgia comes and goes but it can be extremely distressing and may cause serious depression. Fortunately, there is an effective treatment for this particular problem.

Pain is more common in MS than some doctors think. In the past many people were told that pain did not occur, and that if they had pain, MS was not the cause. This is not so and I have come across several people who have experienced severe pain as part of their MS. Once again, I quote from Helen who puts things in her own vivid words.

> I used to have a weird burning pain in my right leg. This was a red-hot flushing sensation coming in waves and rather like a hot cup of tea being poured down my leg – very hot at the top and getting cooler as it trickled down my leg. My leg also felt very tight and weak. This first bout lasted about three weeks.

Sometimes the pain is due to muscle spasms or problems with posture, but often the pain is a sensory disturbance occurring in a particular area of the body.

I remember one lady who came to see me. She described an extremely sensitive pain down one side of her body, causing a problem that was difficult for her to discuss. She was unable to have a normal sexual relationship with her husband because of the pain, and she found it very difficult to talk to him about it, mainly because she was unsure whether the pain was a genuine part of MS. She broke down in tears when I assured her that pain is one of the ways that MS can affect people, and she gained relief from realising that she had a legitimate reason for her sexual difficulties.

Sometimes people have pain due to the postural problems of MS such as back ache; they may get other aches and pains due to being immobile for long periods and remaining too long in one position. There are many examples of pain occurring in MS, and each one needs to be understood and investigated individually so that the right sort of help can be offered.

Pain can sometimes be helped by medication, and a good example of this is the use of Carbamazepine for the treatment of trigeminal neuralgia. This can be very effective, and Carbamazepine can also be used for other pains associated with cranial or peripheral nerves. When drugs do not help in the treatment of pain, some surgical procedures can be effective, and there is also a variety of other techniques that can be used by specialists working in pain clinics. These vary from electrical stimulation to hypnosis and acupuncture. Some people claim that meditation is effective in reducing pain; yoga and other physical methods sometimes seem to help, too.

Spasticity

Spasticity, or involuntary contraction and stiffness of muscles, may affect the arms, legs and trunk. It is common in MS and needs no special treatment unless it is associated with painful spasms or permanent muscle contractures with resulting deformity. Physiotherapy can help by increasing the voluntary control over muscles and by reducing the involuntary spastic contractures (see Chapter 10).

The drugs Baclofen and Diazepam may be used for

treating spasticity, but sometimes they can cause excessive weakness and so may lead to a worsening of disability rather than an improvement. This is because muscle stiffness can actually play a part in helping people to walk when weakness is present. It is important for these reasons not to over-treat spasticity, and each person needs individual assessment before a decision is made by the doctor to use drugs in a particular case.

Diazepam can also cause drowsiness and this limits its use for many people; it may have to be taken at night-time only.

When spasticity, painful spasms, or contractures are severe and have not responded to medicines, then injections into certain nerves can give relief. Sometimes deformity or pain can be dramatically helped by a surgical procedure, when the muscle tendon is cut. But this is only needed by people with severe disability.

Injections around the lower part of the spinal cord can sometimes help those who are confined to bed and who have lost their bladder control. The procedure will result in total paralysis, but it will also lead to the complete loss of painful and deforming spasms in the lower legs. This may sound a drastic action, but for many people it is a price worth paying because they have very little useful power left in their legs, anyway.

Balance and Co-ordination

Sometimes people with MS experience dizzy spells and on these occasions the symptoms of 'nystagmus' may occur. Nystagmus, you might remember, is when the eyes flicker from side to side. I experienced this symptom and found it quite frightening because, as well as the eye problems, I found that whenever I moved my head I felt sick and was unable to stand up without falling over.

Problems of balance are common in MS and many people wobble when they try to stand still. Indeed, there is one particular medical test in which a person is asked to stand up and shut his eyes; if he cannot keep his balance this is an indication that he has lost some of the position sense in his body and that he has been relying on his vision to remain upright. This sign is called 'Romberg's sign', and if a person falls over when he has his eyes shut he is described as being 'Romberg's Positive'.

I have this problem myself and find I have to be especially careful when washing my hair in the shower. As soon as I shut my eyes I tend to fall over! I have solved this problem by having a strong grab-handle in the shower. I now hold onto this until my hair is rinsed free of shampoo and then I can open my eyes and stand upright reasonably steadily.

Demyelination in part of the brain called the cerebellum can cause balance problems and tremor. These symptoms are called 'ataxia' and people with this condition are often quite disabled. Although they still have strength in their arms and legs, they cannot control them properly and the tremor and inco-ordination have disabling affects. There are no effective drugs for loss of balance and co-ordination, but physiotherapy and other remedial treatments can be useful.

The Bladder

As soon as I sat down to write this section I had to get up again to 'have a pee'. This is a frequent occurrence for me (like my father-in-law who has prostate gland trouble) and on 'bad days' it can take me a while to start, a long time to carry out the process in short bursts and then a little while more to decide whether I have really finished. When I decide that I have finished I may have the urge to go again. Then back to work for a while and once again I need to go! (My sister-in-law, Josephine, who is typing this section, tells me that I have described the symptoms of pregnancy! If so, I pity those poor women who have MS and pregnancy at the same time! However, it is worth mentioning that many women who have MS feel much better when they are pregnant, although they might have a temporary exacerbation after the baby is born.)

In MS the bladder is frequently a problem; several different nerves are involved in supplying the muscles of the bladder, and the rings of muscle at the exit are called the 'sphincters'. Demyelination of the spinal cord can therefore lead to complicated urinary symptoms, the most common of which is 'frequency' (having to go to the lavatory very often) and 'urgency' (having to go suddenly). Urgency can also be associated with incontinence, when people cannot hold on to their urine, and this is, of course, socially embarrassing and often leads to people becoming withdrawn and staying at home.

Other people find that their bladder will fill up and will not empty properly. This can eventually lead to a condition called 'retention', when the bladder fills up with urine but the sphincters will not open and let the urine out at all. In these circumstances a person may need to have a tube called a 'catheter' passed into the bladder in order to relieve the pressure and avoid damage to the urinary system.

Bladder difficulties can be helped by various medicines and also by maintaining a high fluid intake to avoid further problems such as infections and the formation of bladder stones. The use of drugs to dampen down over-reactive bladder muscles has not been very encouraging, but the speedy treatment of infections with antibiotics is both effective and very important to keep the kidneys in good health.

When partial incontinence occurs it is wise to develop the habit of emptying the bladder regularly, to avoid constipation, and one should also avoid drinking too much fluid at the wrong times! Intermittent catheterisation, in which a narrow tube is passed into the bladder to empty it properly from time to time, can sometimes help. In a few people, the catheter must be left in place permanently.

When incontinence is a serious problem, electrical stimulation of the spinal cord may be useful, but various surgical procedures are proving to be more effective and are increasingly being used. The idea behind these is to make a way for the urine to come out of the bladder more directly, either through a hole made in the abdomen (an 'urostomy') or by diverting the urine into the intestines.

Many practical domestic aids are available and these, together with specialist information, can be obtained from District Nurses or from the MS Society. These aids include special pads and pants as well as penile sheaths (available to men only!) which divert urine into a bag carried underneath the trousers.

Constipation

Constipation is common in MS due to decreased mobility, weak pelvic muscles and lack of sensation in parts of the bowels. It is therefore important for people with MS to eat plenty of roughage in the diet and to evacuate their bowels regularly in order to prevent constipation occurring. If it is felt that laxatives are needed, it is best to consult a doctor. In severe cases, nursing procedures, such as enemas, may be necessary. Regular exercise, such as swimming or the practice of yoga, can also be beneficial. These, together with a well-balanced diet, are a good way of preventing constipation. As always, prevention is better than cure.

Pressure Sores

These occur easily if someone is immobile and lies or sits in one position for too long. Because sensation is often impaired when a person with MS is immobile, he or she is unable to feel pain and so does not notice when the pressure sores are developing.

For this reason, it is essential for anyone in this situation to be turned or re-positioned frequently and regularly. Sitting in a chair does not mean that 'turning' is unnecessary, because pressure sores can still develop. When a person is immobilised by MS, the community nurse should visit twice a day and extra help will be needed from relatives and friends. Once pressure sores have occurred, admission to hospital is usually necessary; healing can take a long time especially if there are complications, such as an infection.

Single and double water beds are now widely available. They look no different from standard divan beds and I am told that there are even four-poster versions! Water beds distribute pressure evenly and mean that the disabled person does not have to be turned at night. This is an advantage both to the person with MS and to the caring relative.

Peculiar Symptoms

This chapter would be incomplete if I did not mention that many symptoms do not fit neatly into a recognised medical 'pigeon hole', and may seem odd both to the people who have them as well as to those who are trying to help. MS fatigue is dealt with later in the book, but it is worth noting at this point that fatigue can bring on a variety of sensory symptoms which are not normally present. Some of these are difficult to describe, and I know that occasionally people do not like to mention them in case they are laughed at, or thought to be over-imaginative.

Cold legs are sometimes a feature of MS and may be caused by immobility and poor circulation. They may be associated with swollen ankles which can also occur in MS for similar reasons. Alternatively, they might feel cold because of demyelination in the part of the spinal cord which carries the sensory feelings from the legs.

Those who live with a person who has MS, or who are involved in helping, should be aware that unusual or 'funny' symptoms can genuinely occur. It is unpleasant to be ridiculed by someone who fails to take such symptoms seriously or who implies that a big fuss is being made about nothing.

3   Treatment

Because MS is such a variable disease, and because many people experience improvements and remissions for no apparent reason, it is not surprising that there are many claims for many different types of treatment and cure. Unfortunately, none of the so-called cures and few of the treatments have stood either the test of time or the exacting scrutiny of unbiased scientific investigation. Most people have little concept of what scientific proof is all about. They are more likely to decide whether or not a particular treatment is effective from the anecdotes and stories heard from their friends and acquaintances, however bizarre the stories may be. Perhaps the more bizarre the better, because there seems to be a need for dramatic revelation rather than for boring old scientific progress.

In the same way that some people believe that smoking will do no harm because they happen to know an old man of ninety-nine who has 'smoked like a chimney' all his life, there are many people who will believe that a certain diet cures MS because they have read about someone with the disease who made a complete recovery while on the diet. In other words, many people prefer to put their faith blindly into the 'exceptions' rather than the 'rule'.

People with MS frequently have remissions, which can sometimes last a life-time, and there is a natural tendency to seek an explanation for this fact. Many people may not realise that quite dramatic remissions can be a normal part of MS, and if the person who had the remission was receiving 'treatment' at the time, this treatment will be linked with the remission and be regarded as its cause. If they were on a special diet, a particular drug, receiving acupuncture or practising yoga, then the chances are that someone will claim these to be 'cures' for MS. It will become the latest in a long line of 'miracle cures' which are so popular with the Sunday newspapers.

People like to find reasons, and regard the mundane explanation that 'miraculous remissions' are common in MS as being both uninteresting and unlikely. For this reason, proper scientific scrutiny is necessary in order to sift out what is coincidence and what is a genuinely effective treatment.

Treatment Trials

The best way of finding out whether a treatment really works or not is to try it on a large number of people over a period of time and to compare the results with the same number of people, suffering from the same condition, who have not received any treatment at all. It is well known that a large proportion of people will respond for a while to any new treatment, however valuable or valueless it eventually proves to be. People will always feel better if 'something is being done'. This phenomenon is called 'the placebo response' and it must be taken into account in any experiment involving doctors, patients and new treatments.

Other factors that can cause an inaccurate result are the attitudes, beliefs, and enthusiasm (or lack of it) shown by the doctors or scientists carrying out the experiment. They want their particular treatment to work and they may consciously or unconsciously see things as they wish them to be, rather than the way they really are. However well-meaning scientists are, this factor will always play some part. Scientists are human, too, and they want to get results, breakthroughs, be famous; they may even be hoping to win a Nobel Prize!

In order to get over these particular problems, scientists and research workers investigating new treatments have invented the 'multi-centre double-blind controlled trial'.

Quite a mouthful, but an extremely important concept, none the less. What does it mean?

Let us imagine that, as a result of research, a group of scientists consider that substance X could be helpful in alleviating certain symptoms of MS. To find out whether or not this substance does work, doctors and scientists in two or three different 'centres' (hospital or university departments) will set up a treatment trial designed to be as fair and as unbiased as possible.

Each centre will find a number of people who have MS and will divide them into two groups so that each group of people is as similar as possible in terms of severity of the disease, how long they have had MS, sex, age and other such variables. Then one group – 'the subjects', will be given substance X for a period of time while the other group – 'the controls', receives substance Y (which looks exactly like substance X but which is known to be ineffective as a treatment).

The people who actually give the two different treatments to the patients will not know which substance a particular patient is receiving, since the treatments are coded and the codes are held by an independent person. Other independent doctors will regularly examine both the subjects and the controls at each centre throughout the trial. These independent doctors do not know which patients are controls and which are subjects, and they will also keep their own records secret. In this way, neither the patients nor those responsible for giving the 'treatment', nor those who examine and assess the patients' progress, will know who is on which substance. The trial is called 'double blind' because neither the people giving the treatment nor the scientists assessing the response know which patients are having which 'treatments' at any time during the course of the trial.

It is also possible to use a third group of people who are either receiving no 'treatment' at all or else substance Z, and in such cases the same principles will apply. The use of several different centres helps not only by enabling more subjects and controls to be used, but also because it decreases the chance of errors or bias in the experiment, since the experiment is being carried out by several different groups of people at the same time.

At the end of the trial, and after a prearranged period of time, (say two or three years,) the codes are broken and, for the first time, scientists can see just what has happened and whether or not substance X is better than substance Y, or the other way round. If one day a genuine 'miracle cure' were found, the difference between the two groups of patients would quickly become apparent and the codes could be broken earlier if all the scientists agreed.

This is a very complicated process, but it is the only way that unbiased and genuine results about a treatment can be decided. Because of the variability of MS, it is essential to try any new treatment on a large group of people over a long period of time, using all these elaborate safeguards to ensure accuracy. I have spent a lot of time discussing treatment trials because I am sure that if people really understood their value there would be fewer silly arguments and false beliefs about particular treatments.

Sometimes, however, it could be unjustifiable to set up a trial in order to investigate a certain treatment. This might be because the treatment is too dangerous in some way and it is considered unethical to subject people to unnecessary risks without a guarantee of positive result. Another ethical problem could occur when a treatment is already widely accepted as being useful and with few dangers. In this case it might be judged wrong to withhold the treatment from the controls just so as to prove a point that is not generally in dispute, but sadly this problem has not yet arisen with MS.

In the vast majority of situations, the 'double blind controlled trial' technique is not only justifiable but essential. Any treatment which has not been assessed by this process must be regarded with a great deal of suspicion. Although no treatment has yet been proved to cure MS, a few have been shown to be effective either in alleviating some of the symptoms or in speeding recovery from an acute relapse.

Steroids

Steroids are powerful drugs which act by reducing swelling and inflammation in any part of the body. ACTH is a naturally occurring pituitary hormone that stimulates the body itself to produce steroids from the adrenal glands. (It is also known as corticotrophin or as adrenocorticotrophic hormone). It is sometimes prescribed by doctors because controlled clinical trials have shown that it can be effective in shortening the length of acute exacerbations in MS.

ACTH is given in a short course of intramuscular injections and the dose is gradually reduced over a period of three to four weeks. Sometimes steroids are prescribed in tablet form and used in the same way as ACTH. Tablets are more convenient, and possibly just as effective. Both ACTH and steroids (such as Prednisolone) have unpleasant side effects and should not normally be prescribed for long periods, because they can cause unwanted changes in the body, such as high blood pressure. In order to reduce adverse effects steroids are sometimes given intravenously in low doses – but this requires a short stay in hospital.

When I had courses of ACTH, I used to feel very strange at times. Periods of excitement and optimism would alternate with depression, and my sleep pattern was often disrupted. I would like awake for hours at night with my mind racing, and then feel excessively tired during the day.

Being on ACTH also played havoc with my waterworks, and sometimes I would have to go to the loo as many as twelve or more times in a night! Other people with MS tell similar stories. Nevertheless, ACTH and steroids can be effective in relieving unpleasant symptoms and so doctors quite often prescribe them. As is so often the case in medicine, whether or not they will be ultimately helpful will depend on balancing the side effects with the benefits. This will vary from individual to individual, and will therefore require some experimentation in each case.

Other drugs, such as Cyclosporin, influence the immune mechanism by damping down an excessive response, and are being researched. Experiments on another such drug, Cyclophosphamide, have shown that it could benefit some people who have the severe, progressive form of MS. But more work needs to be done in order to ensure that this and similar drugs do not cause more harm than good.

Sunflower and Evening Primrose Oils

There is some evidence that dietary factors could play a part in the development of MS. In particular, it has been shown that increasing the polyunsaturated fats in the diet may be beneficial, leading to an improvement in the clinical course of the disease.

People with MS have been shown to have a lower proportion of linoleic acid in their blood (a polyunsaturated fatty acid) than other people. Two double blind controlled trials have demonstrated that the taking of sunflower seed oil (which is high in linoleic acid) can lead to a small improvement in the course of the disease, with fewer relapses which are also less severe in nature.

(In this typical double blind controlled trial, some people received sunflower seed oil and others received olive oil which was not high in linoleic acid or polyunsaturated fats. Neither the patients nor the doctors knew who had had which oils until after the trial was over and after independent doctors had examined and assessed the subjects for changes in their condition.)

What does this mean for those of us who have MS? We have nothing to lose and will probably benefit from increasing our intake of sunflower seed oil or other foods high in poly-unsaturated fatty acids. We can use sunflower seed oil in salad dressings and cooking; my wife, Penny, uses it to make a very tasty mayonnaise. I also like to add some to mashed potato because you can use quite a lot of oil without noticing the taste too much. There are other oils on the market besides sunflower seed oil which are high in polyunsaturated fatty acids and these are clearly marked.

The recommended dose of sunflower seed oil is 30 mls twice a day (which is equivalent to approximately three tablespoons twice daily). I find that taking sunflower seed oil neat is not pleasant, and I need to keep a small glass of water or, better still, skimmed milk handy to use as a chaser on these occasions. At home we also use margarines which are high in polyunsaturated fats and which are widely available from shops. We spread this on bread and toast and also use it for cooking. I make some quite nice flapjacks using this margarine, but my other cooking abilities are not yet highly developed.

The use of evening primrose oil also has many advocates but so far no controlled trial has shown that it has any value whatsoever. However, some scientists have claimed that, for theoretical reasons, evening primrose oil should be beneficial. I have been taking six capsules of evening primrose seed oil a day for nearly ten years, with no ill effects. I started taking it before the research was published and, being only human, take it just in case I should get worse if I stop! This is, I know, an unscientific and emotional response, and the logical-doctor part of me is quite shocked.

Evening primrose seed oil costs me about eighty pounds a year and, as there is no evidence that it really does help in MS, I cannot legitimately recommend it to other people. The best thing to do is to make up your own mind after studying the evidence for and against. You could read the literature on the subject yourself, but do not be taken in by emotional or anecdotal arguments with no scientific basis. It is a pity that evening primrose seed oil has not been proved to work as it is easier to take than large quantities of sunflower seed oil. On the positive side, I have no hesitation in recommending that you add six tablespoonfuls of sunflower seed oil to your daily diet. Although the results of research are not dramatic, there is at least some evidence that it might help. It is possible to overdo this oil, and some people have put on more weight than they really wanted in such circumstances.

Other Diets

Many other foods, diets and vitamins have been advocated for MS, but there is no evidence that they have any useful part to play. Some can even endanger your health and most of them will make you poorer! The gluten-free diet, in which people are advised to eat nothing which contains wheat flour, such as bread, cakes and biscuits, is one example of a dietary fad that has proved ineffective. Nevertheless, many people still 'believe' in it, despite the evidence that it does no good.

It is important for everyone with MS to eat a healthy diet, and so as well as extra sunflower seed oil, I try to eat as much 'wholefood' as possible. This includes fresh fruit and vegetables and wholemeal bread. More and more, I am beginning to enjoy eating fresh salads and wholewheat pasta, as well as plenty of fresh fruit and yogurt. I have cut down on foods high in saturated fats such as fatty meats, cream, cheese and also some odd items such as avocado pears and coconuts, which may surprise you. I have also cut down on salt and sugar.

I do not consider myself a food faddist (although some of my family might disagree with this) and I also think that at times 'a little of what you fancy does you good'. It is, of course, a good idea to avoid being overweight and to give up smoking if you are able.

Quackery

A large number of people with MS, and often their relatives, too, find it impossible to believe that MS is an incurable illness. They imagine that somewhere there must be a cure, that someone must have the answer to the problem.

It is not a surprising response. It may take most people a long time before they can find the balance between giving in altogether and fighting desperately against the inevitable. We have to go through grief, sadness, shock and anger before we can accept our limits and find new meaning and potential in spite of them.

One stage in this process is to try to deny to ourselves that we have MS, or to pretend that it is not incurable. Because of this we are vulnerable to exploitation; we *want* to believe that there is a diet, cure, treatment that will help us and so we *do* believe it. But perhaps this wishful thinking may also have a positive value. It may lead us to demand more attention for our plight, and thus help to stimulate and promote research. This denial of the truth (for that is really what it is) can therefore be a two-edged weapon. Although it can be effective in getting action, it can also mean that we are victims of quackery.

The press is full of 'breakthroughs' and 'new wonder cures for MS' which usually turn out to be meaningless catch phrases. Magazines, television and radio programmes like to publicise the unusual, the entertaining and the frankly crazy in order to keep their readers and viewers interested. As a result, some people can be left with the mistaken impression that a new diet or treatment for MS has been found which will solve all their problems. This is sad, because spirits and hopes are raised up only to be cruelly dashed when they discover that the media have exaggerated reports of something that, in the end, has no scientific validity.

Following complaints about some of these incidents, several of the more responsible publishers and television producers have become more aware of the danger. They now make sure that they contact the MS Society before they publish, or produce a programme, in order first to check out the facts and make sure that the balance they present is correct. The MS Society is advised by specialists in all fields of research and welfare and they are always available to give advice and talk to the media when required.

However, some people are bound to believe in claims based on the flimsiest of evidence. As I explained earlier, MS is so variable, and so subject to natural improvements and remissions, that anecdotal claims for treatment and cures abound.

The doctors who advise the MS Society look carefully into

any claims that are made and, when it seems justified, an appropriate double blind trial will be set up. Currently trials are going on to establish the truth about Hyperbaric Oxygen therapy. Unfortunately, some people have already jumped to the conclusion that this treatment is effective, on the smallest of evidence. This could be dangerous, since possible adverse long-term effects are as yet unknown and unresearched.

Other current fads are the use of snake venom, mega-vitamins and the gluten-free diet that I mentioned before. Evening primrose seed oil remains controversial and is still an area of continuing research, although there is no evidence at the moment that it has any value.

I occasionally come across people who have resorted to the weirdest of treatments, almost verging on witchcraft, with not even a pseudo-scientific justification behind them. Of course we do all respond, temporarily at least, to novelties and to people who offer us extra attention, and these people can believe, often very sincerely, in what they are doing.

The placebo response is well known to doctors who often use it to boost morale and to give people hope. The use of vitamin B_{12} injections for MS by some doctors falls into this category, as there is no evidence that it will help the disease at all, and despite the fact that B_{12} is readily absorbed if taken by mouth! (I should make it clear that someone who has the uncommon disease, pernicious anaemia, has to be given vitamin B_{12} by injection because in this case it cannot be absorbed by the stomach in the normal way).

I myself was given these injections when I first had MS, but I stopped them as soon as I discovered the truth. How ethical it is for doctors to give placebos is another matter, but when people are demanding treatment, at least they do no harm. This cannot be said for some of the quack treatments offered to the person who has MS. In my experience, relatives can be even more determined to find 'cures' at any cost than the people who actually have MS. Perhaps they feel guilty and are compelled to 'do something' rather than watch someone close to them suffer.

In ancient times it was customary to discredit or even to kill the bearer of bad news. Doctors are often on the receiving end of anger and bitterness from both the patients and the patients' relatives, and they can be unjustly scapegoated. On the other hand, many doctors fail to communicate truthfully with their patients and then doctor-patient relationships can come under a great deal of strain.

When a person is newly diagnosed as having MS she and her relatives often feel confused about the claims for treatment and the various rumours and stories that are told to them about the disease. In these circumstances it is necessary to find out the truth, and there are a number of people who can help. First of all, it is a good idea to discuss the whole area of MS in depth with the family doctor. Many GPs are only too willing to set aside some time in order to help a person or a couple to understand more about the disease and how to live with it. They will also have a reasonably up-to-date knowledge about MS and will be able to give a balanced view on what is a sensible line of approach and what is just quackery. When the family doctor cannot help sufficiently, then the consultant neurologist may be able to answer further questions. Neurologists, however, are spread thinly and many feel that on-going counselling and advice is more appropriate from the GP, health visitor or perhaps from a social worker.

Beta Interferon

Throughout 1995 there was much speculation in the media about this drug, fuelled by the fact that two or three large drug companies began actively to woo the MS world in a way never before observed. Money suddenly became available for an array of new journals and other projects. People with MS were excited by the prospect of an effective treatment for MS backed up by early reports of research projects which, for the first time ever, showed that a significant proportion of people with MS had undoubtedly benefited to some extent when treated with Beta Interferon in controlled trials.

The drug received a licence for the treatment of MS in the UK, but guidance from the NHS Health Executive recommended that it be prescribed by hospital consultants rather than by GPs. Beta Interferon is at present very expensive and I, for one, am not yet convinced that this advice is necessarily in the best interest of MS patients; perhaps it was more about cutting government expenditure? The debate continues and we shall see!

The MS Society, together with other charities involved with MS, has published a useful leaflet about MS and Beta Interferon, based on the story so far. To quote from this leaflet:

> Recent trials do not indicate a cure but show encouraging results for people with relapsing/remitting MS. So far only the results of a trial on mildly affected people have been published and within this group relapses were seen to be reduced by one third. However, these changes have not yet been shown to be accompanied by any significant effect on disability.

All this is very positive and there is no doubt that progress is being made quite quickly now. But caution is needed – some top neurologists are unconvinced that Beta Interferon really is as good as early results seemed to indicate, and there are also reports of some adverse effects from the drug. A lot more research needs to be carried out, but if you want to see if Beta Interferon might help you or someone close to you, talk to the doctor and check out the latest advice from the MS charities.

4 Diagnosis and Doctors

Many people with MS are dissatisfied with the way that they have been treated by their doctors. Quite often they express strong feelings of bitterness, anger or disillusion. Perhaps this is not so surprising in the light of a recent survey which showed that a large number of people with MS had not been told by their family doctors that they had the disease and that most of them resented this.

Because I have MS myself I am able to understand these feelings. I am also a doctor and so I belong to both camps, and I do not pretend to be objective or detached in my outlook. On the contrary, I am emotionally involved and my views result from living with my own MS as well as from helping others through counselling and working as a psychiatrist. In this double role I have benefited from hearing confidences from people with MS which they would not usually share with their doctors. I have also been able to listen to the ideas and anxieties that my doctor friends have expressed about their patients.

MS often leads to a long and complicated illness, and there are many different occasions when help and understanding from a physician are needed. Particularly stressful for families are the occurrences of frightening relapses and complications. Incontinence, bedsores, or the need to depend on aids for the first time, can all cause emotional and relationship difficulties as well as physical ones. When sexual problems occur, whether for physical or psychological reasons, or from a mixture of the two, then skilled counselling from a doctor is essential, as well as a knowledge of the disease and its many manifestations. Families also need time, support and information when pregnancy is an issue, or when long- or short-term residential care is being considered.

The Diagnosis

A most important time, when a doctor's skill is often tested to the limit, is the time of diagnosis. Poor communication of a definite or suspected diagnosis is responsible for as much distress, misunderstanding and ill-feeling as at any other period in the relationship between doctor and patient. The diagnosis of MS may be difficult to make, depending as it does on a pattern of symptoms and signs occurring over a period of time. There are still no really reliable diagnostic tests for MS and the disease is often suspected before it can be confirmed by subsequent events. But an early diagnosis is desirable to exclude other, treatable conditions and to meet the needs of research into the disease. Equally important are the emotional needs of the person with MS and of his or her family who are faced with the frightening experience to which they must adjust before they can plan the future. Honesty from the doctor will enhance the doctor/patient relationship and will eventually lead to a greater trust in him or her by the patient.

Early Symptoms

The diagnosis of MS depends, firstly, on obtaining a clear history from the patient. If MS is present, some people will complain of symptoms which fit into a pattern characteristic of the disease, and in these cases the diagnosis will be fairly straightforward. In MS, scars (called plaques or sclerosis) are scattered throughout the central nervous system; these have been caused by attacks of inflammation and loss of 'white matter' (myelin). This process is called 'demyelination' and the loss of this myelin, which surrounds many nerve fibres, results in a slowing down or a complete absence of impulses along the nerves affected. Symptoms of MS are due to the damage caused by demyelination occurring in *different places* in the brain and spinal cord at *different times*. It is this pattern of symptoms occurring in different places (dissemination in space) and at different times (dissemination in time) which is so characteristic of MS and gave rise to the old name disseminated sclerosis.

In the early stages of the disease, as I have described, the attacks usually cause well-defined symptoms which then get better quite quickly over a few days, weeks or months, leaving little or no disability. Supposing someone has a history of blurred vision and pain in one eye and then a few months or a few years later complains of weakness in a leg. The doctor will observe that the two symptoms have occurred separated in time and in different parts of the central nervous system. MS should be suspected and, if further symptoms develop, such as clumsiness in an arm, or a loss of sensation down the front of a leg, then the diagnosis can be made with confidence, needing very little further investigation.

Difficult Problems

About one in five people with MS do not have a relapsing and remitting pattern of symptoms. They may complain instead of symptoms which have come on gradually and with no recovery periods. This is likely to happen in the sort of MS which mainly affects the spinal cord and which first shows itself in middle-aged people who have a progressive weakness in both legs.

Other diagnostic difficulties can arise if the symptoms are vague, transient or poorly defined. They can seem like the symptoms of anxiety or depression and may be dismissed by the doctor as unimportant, or as a reason for prescribing tranquillisers or antidepressant drugs. MS symptoms of this sort include fatigue, dizzy spells, strange sensations, pins and needles, difficulty in concentration and loss of memory.

Sometimes people wonder why they have to wait a long time before a diagnosis of MS can be made when they have a symptom on its own, such as weakness in one leg, for which no other cause can be found. This is because one symptom on its own, even if it appears typical of MS, must not be diagnosed as MS without a very good reason. It is also important that the doctor should exclude treatable conditions like certain brain or spinal tumours as the cause of the symptoms. A diagnosis of MS must only be made if there is no evidence of any other possible cause of the symptoms, and there must be evidence that areas of damage in the brain and spinal cord are scattered both in time and in space.

Investigations
Because it is often difficult to make a positive diagnosis from the medical history alone, doctors may use laboratory tests and other investigations to help them reach a conclusion. None of these investigations in itself will point directly to MS, but taken together they can help to exclude other conditions, and indicate that MS could be a strong possibility.

The first of these tests is the examination of the cerebrospinal fluid (CSF) that bathes the brain and the spinal cord. This is extracted by a simple procedure called a lumbar puncture (LP) and the fluid is analysed for changes in the amount and type of protein present. An increase in the white blood cells or a typical change in the protein pattern would support a diagnosis of MS, but other types of change in the CSF would give reason to think of an alternative cause of the problem.

Another test frequently used is the visual evoked response (VER). The patient is asked to look at a chequer board or a flashing light and the time taken for the message from the eyes to reach the back of the brain (occipital cortex) is measured using special electrodes attached to the scalp. If there is a delay, so that the message takes longer than usual to reach the occipital cortex, then it is probable that demyelination has occurred in the optic nerves. Since the optic nerves are often affected in MS, even when there are no visual symptoms noticed by the patient, evidence of this kind can be very important in doubtful cases. If there is no evidence of a delay in the VER, it does not rule out a diagnosis of MS, but it might perhaps mean that the patient should have another investigation called a 'myelogram'. This is done in order to exclude a spinal tumour, which might be the real cause of symptoms such as weakness or loss of sensation in the legs. (A myelogram is a special sort of X-ray of the spinal cord in which some of the CSF is replaced by a substance which acts as a contrast, so making it easier to see any abnormalities in the spinal cord.)

Brain scans can also show up MS plaques, but until recently they have not shown sufficient detail and their use has been limited. An exciting new development is the nuclear magnetic resonance scanner (MRI scanner) which can make detailed images of nearly all parts of the inside of the body. Instead of using potentially harmful radiation (as in X-rays), it uses a harmless magnetic field and radio waves. The MRI scanner is likely to revolutionise the diagnosis of MS in the future, but it will take some while for it to be generally available. It may soon be possible to make the diagnosis of MS on the first occasion that a symptom arises, but this is not yet feasible and much more research and development is needed first.

Another diagnostic test currently being researched is whether the movement of red or white blood cells in an electrical field is different in people who have MS from those who do not have the disease, or who have some other neurological condition. So far the evidence is insufficient to form any definite conclusion and tests based on this idea have not yet been accepted by the medical profession as having a useful role to play in diagnosis.

Telling the Truth
There is a great deal of argument surrounding the issue of 'telling the patient', and many people with MS have claimed that they were not told the truth in a straightforward manner. Some have found out by accident, while others have had to resort to subterfuge, such as steaming open doctors' letters or reading hospital notes upside down. Sometimes a wife has been informed of the diagnosis but instructed not to tell her partner who actually has the disease. Inevitably, this places a great strain on family relationships.

Even when the diagnosis is certain, a doctor's reluctance to tell may be justified on the grounds that the person cannot cope with the knowledge. Yet time after time, people with MS speak of relief at knowing their diagnosis, just as I did myself when my own MS was finally confirmed. Naturally, many are shocked and distressed, but at least they know the truth and can begin to come to terms with it; the truth is rarely worse than the unknown.

An American study found that a great deal of conflict arises between MS patients and physicians during the period before a diagnosis is made. Many patients begin to take an active part in discovering their own diagnosis and it was found that these conflicts extended to relationships with family and friends. However, 'naming the disease' resulted in a reduction of stress and the investigators urged doctors to consider these emotional factors when deciding whether or not to inform patients of a suspected diagnosis of MS.

Understanding the Doctor

But what about the doctors? We need to understand them, too! In these modern times of 'high tech' medicine, doctors may feel trained *to cure* rather than *to care* for their patients. It sometimes seems that medical students are chosen for their ability to pass examinations rather than for their more human qualities. Medical training may perpetuate this bias and doctors may come to see their role as technical experts in the diagnosis and treatment of disease. They may prefer to see quick and positive results and may only feel that they have succeeded if a patient gets better. While being useful in some medical conditions, this approach can leave a doctor feeling less confident when faced with the vague and recurrent symptoms of long-term illness. More particularly, he or she may find it difficult to cope with the emotional side of the disease.

Technical expertise and medical knowledge, although essential, are not enough. In order to be wholly effective, a doctor must combine these with communication and counselling skills. A balance between bedside manner and technical competence is needed today, just as it was at the end of the sixteenth century when Francis Bacon wrote in an essay, 'Physicians are some of them so pleasing and conformable to the humour of the patient as they press not the true cure of the disease; and some others are so regular in proceeding according to art for the disease, as they respect not sufficiently the condition of the patient. Take one of middle temper. . . .'

The doctor must also be able to cope with his or her own feelings of inadequacy or frustration when faced with an MS patient, and must not take personally any unreasonable anger and bitterness projected on to him or her. It is most important that doctors should realise that they can help their patients by giving them time and interest and, on occasions, by 'just listening'. We can all gain a great deal of relief when sharing our fears and confused feelings, and by being accepted as human beings and not just 'patients'.

Patients or People?

Throughout the world, people with MS dislike being referred to as MS patients, MS persons, multiple sclerotics or 'MSers'. Persons with Multiple Sclerosis International (PWMSI) have recommended that all such labels be dropped and that we are always referred to as people or persons with multiple sclerosis. I am very much in favour of this general rule but feel that the word patient is still acceptable and necessary if limited to those occasions when a person with MS is consulting or being treated by his or her doctor. I have tried to follow this rule in my book but inevitably there will be border-line cases, and I know that I am unlikely to please everyone!

The Doctor as Scapegoat

Once we have been diagnosed as having MS, we must live with a disease which is both humiliating and depressing. We have to cope with loss of health and security, as well as changed roles in the family and at work, which may be devastating to our self-respect. People can feel angry and may look for someone to blame. Many are so eager to find an explanation and cure that they turn to quack remedies or diets. In both these circumstances the doctor will be the natural scapegoat and may be rejected or treated unfairly. Unfortunately, at this point some doctors are upset by the patient's reaction and may feel unable to cope with the relationship. The outcome of this may be that the doctor does not wish to see the patient more than he has to, or may pass him or her on to someone else.

Invisible Symptoms

As well as coming to terms with loss, the person with MS has to cope with the vague initial symptoms of the disease which are subjective but very real. These symptoms are often difficult to describe without appearing to be 'neurotic' or a 'hypochondriac'. Such labels are sometimes used by doctors, but they serve only to undermine the trust and goodwill in the relationship between the patient and the doctor. Visual or sensory symptoms, and in particular MS fatigue, are hard for patients and close relatives to understand. It is important that doctors give reassurance and an explanation so that everyone understands that the person with MS really is ill. Because of the difficulties involved in communicating symptoms, a person may deny or hide them; others may exaggerate the symptoms, often in an emotional way, and so encourage the doctor's suspicion that they are 'purely psychological'. Both these behaviours inevitably lead to a further breakdown in communication.

The Doctor's Dilemma - How Much to Tell

Some doctors think that it is not always in the best interests of MS patients to be told the truth at an early stage, or even to be told the truth at all. They argue that the doctor's first duty is the relief of suffering and that to tell the truth could cause unnecessary anguish rather than peace of mind. They will point out that a patient presenting early in the course of the disease and having had only two or three MS symptoms, could be free from further illness for many years or even for a life-time. Another justification for deceiving people about the possible outcome is that it is impossible to predict the future with certainty, and that patients are not able to understand the complexities involved.

Not knowing whether a patient really wants to face the truth can be a good reason for being cautious about how much to tell. But dishonesty justified on these grounds sometimes results from the doctor's own discomfort when discussing emotionally painful issues. The doctor's unconscious anxiety could be the real cause for not being truthful, rather than a genuine regard for the patient's needs.

A few people with MS have told me that they resented being given their diagnosis early because they had altered family and career plans unnecessarily in the light of subsequent events. In these cases the failure could have been in *how* they were told rather than *how much* they were told. A gloomy picture of the future may have been given by a doctor with a pessimistic view of the disease based on treating severely disabled patients in hospital. But many people with MS live normal lives and may have little or no disability for many years.

In my experience, the vast majority of people with MS have wanted to know the nature of their disease as early as possible. They have been keen to discover all that they could about MS to enable them to make their own decisions about the future. Many have felt that they had a right to know about their own illness and to control their own treatment.

A moral question for the doctor is whether to do what he or she thinks is right when this differs from the patient's wishes. It is difficult for the doctor to be sure that he or she accurately knows what the patient really wants. Although there are no simple answers to these questions, they emphasise the need for the doctor not just to understand the patient, but also to be aware of his or her own attitudes. He or she must be prepared to consider what the truth could mean for a particular patient, and it is surely right to respect a person's need to make his or her own decisions. The doctor's prime task must be to serve the patient and the patient's family and to provide them with the information and support that they require to adapt to the demands of an uncertain future.

Information and Support

Can communication between doctor and patient be improved? Telling someone a disturbing diagnosis or prognosis is not just a question of the transfer of information, but of establishing an appropriate relationship. It is difficult to take in more than a little information in the clinical atmosphere of the consulting room at a time of emotional shock. People often forget what they have been told under these conditions and may sometimes deny that they have been given a diagnosis at all!

Diagnosing MS is not just about informing people of the facts, but about being sensitive to their emotional needs and reacting appropriately to them. It is often best for a patient and close relative to be seen together, for as long as they need, to ask questions and to express their feelings. Opportunities must be provided for them to return for more information and support, and time is necessary for people to work through their feelings of shock, fear, anger and sadness at each stage of the disease. Some people need to deny part of the truth until they can cope with it all, and skill is needed to assess how much someone really wants to know at any one time. The truth should not be forced on people any more than it should be withheld completely.

Who Should Tell?

A question often discussed by those of us who have MS is whether the neurologist or the general practitioner is the best person to inform a patient that he has the disease. Each case is unique and will depend on the circumstances surrounding it.

It is often appropriate for a neurologist to tell someone that he has MS, or to discuss suspicions that this might be so, and I know that many see this as their responsibility. But this will only be satisfactory if the neurologist can offer the patient and family the chance to be seen on several occasions. Only such an approach will allow them to question the neurologist, work through their feelings and obtain the necessary emotional support, as well as information. In many cases it will be the GP who has the time and skills necessary, especially if, as the family doctor, he or she has already established a relationship with the patient.

Whatever is decided by the doctors, it is essential that GPs and neurologists work closely together, and are absolutely clear about their individual responsibilities. Unfortunately this is not always so, and patients may find themselves cast adrift between the 'devil and the deep blue sea'.

The Family

When one member of the family has MS, the whole family will be affected; children can be very sensitive to anxiety and may become disruptive and attention-seeking if their needs are ignored. Facts should be explained to them and, if they are involved in major family decisions, they will not feel excluded and resentful.

The process of grieving that surrounds loss of health and future security may last a long time. Patients and relatives will need to express their natural feelings and this can be painful for those working or living with them. If this process is blocked, there is a risk that personal and relationship difficulties can occur, requiring psychiatric help at a later stage.

'Telling the truth' to the patient and relatives is basically a counselling exercise, requiring an understanding of psychological processes, self-awareness and relationship skills. But the doctor does not always have sufficient time or the required training. Often a nurse or a social worker will be able to help on these occasions and may be in a better position to provide the regular follow-up that is so necessary when a diagnosis of MS has been made. For this to happen, there must be a shared understanding of each other's roles by all involved, as well as mutual trust and respect.

The Patient's Responsibility

Patients also have a responsibility to communicate with the doctor. Doctors are not mind readers and they cannot guess what is worrying their patients unless the patients ask questions and state their fears. Sometimes someone with long-standing MS can become an expert in the disease and may be disillusioned with a doctor who has only limited experience. This puts a strain on the relationship, but it is unfair to expect a GP to know everything about MS when he or she may only have one or two patients with the disease in the practice. People working for the MS Society can also become frustrated with a local doctor for similar reasons.

Some doctors are prepared to admit lack of complete knowledge about MS and to acknowledge the possible expertise of MS patients. One lady told me that her GP's reaction to a note from a consultant neurologist, confirming the diagnosis of MS, was to share the letter with her and say, 'I don't really know much about MS: let's find out what we can together.' And that is exactly what they have been doing ever since, with great benefit to them both, I am sure! Similarly, another doctor, when dealing with complications of MS, said to his patient, 'You're the expert, tell me what you know about this problem and I'll do my best to help.'

These encouraging responses are rather different from the reply given to another person who asked whether it might be useful to meet someone else with MS. The doctor, in this case a consultant neurologist, answered, 'Don't be so silly! The next thing that you will be doing is writing to the MS Society for leaflets.' Unhelpful responses like this are all too common, and I hear reports of this kind quite regularly, both in Britain and from overseas.

People with MS and their families can learn to share responsibility with the doctors for their medical care and treatment. The doctor/patient relationship has been compared with that of the elephant and the mahout (elephant driver). The elephant is a strong, powerful and useful creature but, if not managed properly, can become dangerous for those very reasons. It is essential that the mahout makes sure that the elephant does not roll over, or sit in the wrong places, and that a group of elephants are not accidentally stampeded!

Similarly, the patient has to manage 'the medical advisers' if he is to get the best out of them. For this partnership to be effective, both the doctors and patients must make a positive effort to understand and respect each other.

Improving Communication

There are ways in which we can help to dispel some of the misunderstanding that exists between the doctor and the person who has MS. First, we must clearly define to the medical profession the special psychological needs of people with MS. In particular, we should express our dissatisfaction with the low priority given to counselling skills at all levels of medical education. People who have MS can be difficult to deal with, but it is ultimately the doctor's responsibility to overcome problems and to understand that they are often due to the person's response to a frightening and confusing disease. Indeed, sometimes the disease itself can cause direct psychological symptoms which may include memory loss, irritability, mood swings and, in severe cases, dementia.

Secondly, MS Societies can try to compensate for the lack of counselling available by training their own personnel to cope better with psychological problems by acquiring their own counselling skills. Giving advice or providing aids and holidays, whilst important, is certainly not enough. Some people who have MS could be trained as counsellors and the further development of self-help groups, which have been so successful in the past few years, could be encouraged. Indeed, this is already happening in some places.

Thirdly, we can all support people better in standing up to

their doctors and making their needs clearly known. We can encourage them to ask more questions and to complain if they are not satisfied with the service that they are getting. Perhaps there could be more meetings between professionals and volunteer helpers; MS Societies have an important role to play in this area, and I would like to see local groups taking more responsibility for liaison with the medical profession.

The emotional and social difficulties experienced by families with MS very often cause more pain and suffering than the physical effects of the disease. People who have been diagnosed as having MS, as well as those who wish to help them, need to understand these emotional factors more fully. Communication will only improve when doctors and those they are trying to help become free from the fears and prejudices that so often seem to complicate their relationships. In the last resort, it is always possible to change to another doctor.

5 Fatigue and Psychological Problems

Everybody, fit or ill, experiences fatigue, but for people with MS it has a special significance. Whereas, for most people, it is caused by tiredness and weakness affecting muscles after exercise or exertion, in the case of many people with MS it also involves the nervous system.

The cause of MS fatigue is not fully understood. What may happen is that it becomes more difficult for the nerve impulses to travel along the demyelinated nerves, so that the strength of the impulses is much reduced. Sensory nerves as well as motor nerves can cause weakness, a tired heavy feeling of muscles, inco-ordination and shakiness. Fatigue of sensory nerves, which help us to see, hear, taste and smell, and enable us to distinguish how objects feel, can cause problems in one or more of these senses. When we are fatigued, we do not just experience a heaviness, we may also have blurred vision, numbness, or other difficulties in the sensory system.

While fatigue in MS may be brought on by exertion, it can also occur for other reasons. It has been discovered that it can be caused by eating a heavy meal, by smoking and by hot temperatures; for example, having a hot bath. This last experience is so common that a 'hot bath test' has been developed for MS.

Many people who have MS feel much worse after a hot bath, and may experience blurred vision, general weakness and increased difficulty in walking. Most feel better when cool but some claim that they are more fatigued when they are cold. The extra symptoms that occur after a hot bath, or when fatigued, are temporary, and no long-term harm will result.

Our body temperature fluctuates over a twenty-four hour period and is about one degree F° more in the afternoons than in the early mornings. Because of this, many with MS are most fatigued in the late afternoon and may need to take a rest at this time.

Fatigue after exertion can be an early feature of MS, as I found, and I remember also that when I first developed the disease I had pain in my left eye with a strange feeling in the corner of my vision. I kept looking up but there was nothing there. Old symptoms may return if you are fatigued. If you have been exercising or having a hot bath, you may find that symptoms experienced during a previous relapse come back. Sometimes you may wonder whether you are having another attack. I once had a very late night, and when I lay down to go to sleep, I had severe vertigo. I thought, 'Oh no, not another relapse!' It wasn't. I was just very tired, and it was the effect of fatigue. It soon cleared up.

MS fatigue seems to happen faster than ordinary fatigue. For instance, if I begin to dig the garden, I start off well but about three or four minutes later I feel very tired indeed. I used to wonder what the devil was going on, and my wife thought that I was trying to get out of the work! If I hadn't had MS, I should have been able to dig the garden for about an hour before fatigue was experienced. Recovery from MS fatigue also takes much longer than from ordinary fatigue. When I have had a hot bath or too much exercise, I have to lie down for at least half an hour before I recover.

Some people find that their speech becomes worse after exertion or being overheated, or fatigue may cause tingling in the hands and feet, like pins and needles. It varies very much from individual to individual, so one person with MS may have much less fatigue after exertion or hot baths than another.

Fig 3 illustrates how signs and symptoms are exaggerated after exertion, overheating or infection. Triangle A represents the 'before' and Triangle B represents the 'after'. The tip of Triangle A indicates the 'signs' that can be detected by the

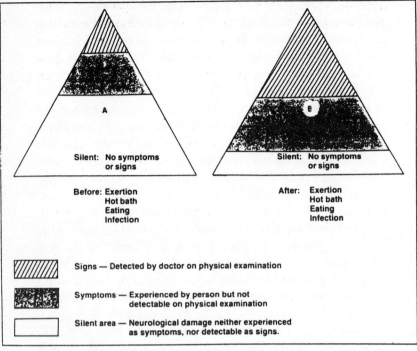

Fig 3. Characteristics and effects of MS fatigue, showing how symptoms are exacerbated by specific events.

neurologist when he or she examines you (reflexes that are exaggerated or inverted, weakness, poor co-ordination). The middle section represents the 'symptoms' you yourself feel – heaviness in a limb; blurring of vision; tingling in fingers. There may be no corresponding signs that the neurologist can find. (I began to lose faith in neurologists to some extent, because they often told me there was nothing wrong with me, and that my symptoms would completely disappear. I was assured several times that my vision was normal, but I knew subjectively that it wasn't. I was also assured that the tingling sensation would disappear from my hand, which it hasn't completely.)

At the bottom of the triangle is a large section labelled 'silent area'. This stands for the damage to the nerve insulating area, the myelin. A lot of demyelination takes place in our brains and spinal cord when we have MS without necessarily producing any symptoms or signs; so the silent area represents myelin damage that, for the moment, is causing neither symptoms we feel nor signs that a neurologist can detect.

Triangle B illustrates what happens after exertion or after a hot bath. The person now experiences more of the neurological damage caused by the disease. He or she may feel much weaker and more tired, and vision may become worse. Pins and needles can occur, as well as a depressing feeling of fatigue, rather like having the 'flu.

The symptom area of Triangle B is accordingly much greater and illustrates why the hot bath test is useful in testing for multiple sclerosis. If you feel there is something wrong with you, but don't show any neurological signs on examination, you might be given the hot bath test. If signs show up after the bath, the neurologist can then say, 'Yes, there are signs of MS. There is neurological damage.'

As you can see, the silent area is still there, but is smaller than before. The person is experiencing the damage that exists in the silent area, but which does not ordinarily show up. Indeed, in some people the signs and symptoms of multiple sclerosis remain silent throughout their entire lives. A Swiss pathologist discovered, by doing post-mortems on a large number of people, that about one in five of those with MS had not been diagnosed clinically. No one, including the people themselves, knew they had MS. If their conditions were illustrated by a triangle, you would just see a large silent area. Perhaps, when they were fatigued or ill, some slight symptoms may have been present, but possibly no signs ever showed up. Some of them may have been diagnosed as having a condition other than MS.

To summarise, when we become fatigued, we have a shift downwards in the triangle. We become more aware of the symptoms, and the signs of the disease become more obvious to an observer.

Problems Caused by Fatigue in MS

Unfortunately, having fatigue can cause a lot of problems - physical, psychological, family and social. Physical problems are perhaps the most obvious at first. For instance, if you are a manual labourer you can't do the same job without getting very tired and exhausted. Fatigue may cause problems in other parts of your life as well. It may be more difficult to look after children who are young and active; it may be impossible for your sex life to continue in quite the same way as before.

Psychological problems can develop if an early diagnosis is not obtained. People wonder what these strange feelings are that they have when they are tired. They wonder why the symptoms occur, why the doctor says there is nothing wrong with them, and why, after they have been to the doctor several times, he or she seems to suggest that they are neurotic! It can happen that people who have MS are labelled as having psychiatric problems in the early stages. In some cases, MS may not progress beyond the feeling of tiredness or blurred vision and may, therefore, never be diagnosed.

Even after the disease has been diagnosed, it is difficult for family doctors to understand the subjective side, the symptoms that we feel. Neurologists see more people with MS than general practitioners do, but they don't see them regularly, and they don't get to know them as people. Therefore, for different reasons neurologists may also fail to distinguish what is fatigue and what is a reaction to having a chronic illness like MS - a feeling of depression or anxiety.

People with MS are often depressed and worried about what is happening. This is a natural reaction, but unfortunately, the symptoms of anxiety and depression are similar to those of fatigue. You experience heaviness, a lack of energy, a feeling of tiredness. Who is to say what is depression and anxiety and what is MS? It is extremely difficult to tell, as I myself found out when I experienced all these things at once. The result is that, the more depressed you become, the more you wonder what is going on. Until you have sorted it out with help and understanding – perhaps by talking it over with someone else who has MS – you have to deal with a lot of anxiety. I think one of the values of self-help groups is to enable people with MS to share their experiences. After talking to others, they often feel relieved and know that their feelings are normal; they are not the psychiatric cases they feared themselves to be!

Many people with MS have told me that friends or relatives have remarked on their fit and healthy appearance. 'Are you sure that you have MS? You look so well.' Often, on these occasions, the person with MS has been feeling awful, and these comments can leave him angry, hurt and misunderstood. He may also feel guilty and respond apologetically, or even deny altogether his true awareness of being ill.

I mentioned that problems can occur in relationships because of fatigue. In my case, Penny (my wife) complained I was trying to get out of doing the gardening. I had fatigue which I couldn't understand or accept, so I would persist in trying to garden but then find out that I just had to sit or lie down for a while. When we talked to other people with MS, we discovered that what was happening was normal. Now we make allowances. She does the practical, manual things about the house, and I do paperwork and things which don't require so much physical effort. We have adjusted: I have changed my role, and she has changed hers. I think it is very important that the role changes be tackled head on, and that people be encouraged to change roles realistically. This requires understanding by all members of the family, not just the person who has MS.

Role changes also apply to sexual activity. If the more sexually assertive partner develops MS, it may be necessary for the other person to become more active. Otherwise, their enjoyment of sexual relations may be impaired and may completely stop. It may even cause marriage breakdown if they misunderstand each other. The partner without MS may think the other one isn't interested any more. A lot of problems relating to the sexual side of life occur in healthy people, so it is not surprising that people who have MS experience them as well.

What Can be Done to Help?

In relieving the effects of fatigue, I think it is most important to *understand*, to realise that fatigue does occur, and that it is an integral part of having MS. It is important not only for us to understand it, but also for our relatives and our employers to understand and to help us make adjustments in our lifestyle. It is important to express our feelings and our worries, and to talk with other people with MS who have experienced fatigue so that we can work out how it affects us. I think it is also important that those in the 'health care professions', such as nurses, doctors, physiotherapists and occupational therapists, should understand fatigue. They must appreciate that MS can cause fatigue which may show up to varying degrees in different people. Therefore, education for health care professionals must continue.

I think it is essential that we remain physically fit. We can't do much about our damaged nerves, except to avoid hot baths, but we can keep fit within the scope of our physical abilities. While you would probably not expect me to advocate athletics – running, for instance – you can get exercise in other ways. It must not be overdone, but it must be sufficient to keep you in good condition. Each person should arrange a balanced programme that suits his or her preferences – swimming, yoga, callisthenics, whatever. I have found that the best routine for me is to exercise fairly strenuously twice a day and follow the sessions with a short rest. Physical fitness will be enhanced by following a sensible diet and giving up smoking or losing weight if necessary.

You must plan your work routine, your social occasions and your late nights so that they don't all come in a row. Unfortunately, it doesn't always work out very well in practice, and I sometimes find I am going out every night of the week. I realise I am in danger of causing a relapse, but sometimes it is very difficult to plan ahead. But we do need willpower, and we must be able to say 'no'. Moderation must be the word, so that you don't overdo, and yet don't opt out and underdo.

There are some specific activities, as well, that we can use to deal with fatigue. Physiotherapy can help people regain the use of muscles after a relapse. Co-ordination exercises are also important. Yoga, too, can be helpful; it is a form of physiotherapy, but it is also a form of training, a discipline. One of the main principles of yoga is that you never do anything beyond your capability. It is completely non-competitive. You go to your own limit and no more, and therefore it is ideally tailored for people who have MS. To quote a woman who has been involved with yoga for some time:

I know, of course, that yoga will not restore nerves and muscles which have been irreparably damaged by MS, but it is certainly helping me to maintain a better standard of general health than previously, and the breathing exercises and relaxation have resulted in a calmer state of mind and a happier outlook. Yoga has given me a new interest in life, and also introduced me to a new circle of faces and kind, friendly people.

That explains it exactly. Yoga doesn't do anything to nerves which have been damaged, but it is one way of keeping fit, and by joining a group, you make sure you receive regular exercise. I shall deal more fully with the subject of yoga and MS in a later chapter.

Yoga combined with a rest/exercise programme of a more traditional sort could be a good way of planning one's life. It is part of my day. I don't pretend to be a paragon of virtue, but every morning I spend about four minutes doing press-ups and yoga, and I do another four minutes in the evening. That is only eight minutes a day, but I do it every day and if you add it up over a month, it is quite a lot of exercise. The important thing is not the length of time, but the regularity.

An additional benefit of regular exercise, some people report, is the reduction of muscle spasms. Spasms occur when a muscle goes into a strong contraction and doesn't relax. It can be quite painful. In some people they occur when they are fatigued, so by following a regular regime of exercise and rest, they are able to avoid this particular complication. Certain medicines can also help prevent muscle spasms.

In conclusion, although fatigue is very much a symptom of multiple sclerosis, it is one that can be managed, if understood. Fatigue may be experienced as overwhelming tiredness (lassitude) or as sensory difficulties – blurred vision, slurred speech, pins and needles, numbness. Fatigue may be brought on by exertion, heat, infection or overeating. When fatigue is experienced, the signs and symptoms of MS become more pronounced. Unless fatigue is recognised and understood, people who have MS may be thought by their families, friends and employers to have psychological problems. Talking with others who have MS is a good way to understand the problems fatigue can cause and to learn methods of overcoming them. A regular exercise programme is helpful in becoming and staying fit. Moderation is the key to leading a full and happy life, but occasionally, extremes give spice.

Invisible Symptoms

For people who do not have MS, fatigue is perhaps the most difficult symptom to understand, but there are many other symptoms that are invisible, although very real to the person who experiences them. In my own case, I often feel that people do not really understand that I have blurred vision and blind spots in both eyes, together with a fading of the colour red. They often suggest that I need spectacles and it is remarkably difficult trying to explain how my visual defects have arisen, and that my eyes themselves are perfectly normal. The damage has occurred in my optic nerves which lie between my eyes and my brain, and even the strongest of glasses would make no difference!

I have also experienced numbness and loss of position sense in my arm. This has caused me to spill coffee over myself, and others, and to behave in a clumsy manner which is very embarrassing. Another invisible symptom that I have already described is related to my bladder. There are times when I go to the lavatory very often, sometimes in quick succession, and there are other times when I have to go quite suddenly. This can prove a problem if I am staying overnight away from home. I worry in case my constant chain-pulling wakes up my hosts! I have to face the dilemma of whether to pull the chain or to risk others in the house coming across a smelly and unflushed lavatory as the price they pay for a quiet night.

Many people with MS will experience unpleasant sensations of pain which vary in type from person to person and I have dealt with this subject already. Certainly, having invisible symptoms can cause much embarrassment, annoyance and even anguish; other people receive more sympathy for a cold or a sprained ankle!

Psychological Symptoms

The medical profession has traditionally associated MS with the symptom of 'euphoria'. This means a feeling of well-being and happiness which is in contrast to the severity of the illness, and it implies that the person concerned is unaware of the serious nature of his or her condition. I remember that, as a medical student, I was told that this euphoria was a great blessing for the patients, since it compensated for the otherwise cruel nature of the disease.

Euphoria is still thought to occur frequently in people who are severely disabled with MS, but it is now recognised that depression is a much more serious and common problem. Indeed, people who at first appear euphoric often turn out, on deeper examination, to be seriously depressed.

It is not surprising that many people with MS are depressed by what is a frightening and often progressive disease. Much of the depression that occurs is understandable in terms of the experience of natural grief; it would be odd if we did not feel sad and angry about our MS.

However, some people with MS experience a deep and very long-lasting depression which does not respond to counselling and may require psychiatric treatment, possibly with the use of antidepressant medicines. This depression is thought to be directly associated with neurological damage and it is therefore part of the disease process. Rarely, MS first shows as a depressive illness or other psychiatric problem, and the physical effects of the disease may only emerge later.

Memory Loss and Mood Swings

Not uncommonly, people with MS find that they lose some control over their feelings; they may cry or laugh for little reason and they may become frightened of over-reacting in front of others. This is embarrassing and may lead to social withdrawal and isolation. Sometimes rapid mood swings will occur and a person can appear happy and then sad in quick succession. This is not only confusing to the person concerned, but also to his or her family and friends. I remember talking to a man with MS who was about thirty-five years old; he said that he was extremely concerned because sometimes, for no real reason, he would start to laugh and when he laughed he could not stop. Inside he felt very foolish and upset, and in fact he was suffering from a deep depression; eventually he made a suicide bid.

Quite often people who have MS experience problems with memory and concentration. These cause a lot of worry, both for the person who has the problems and for his family, leading to misunderstanding and frustration.

These difficulties can occur at any stage of the disease and are not necessarily related to how far the person is disabled in other ways. I have often found that people in the very early stages of MS complain of loss of memory and are quite concerned about whether or not it is part of the disease. It is helpful to realise that these are true symptoms of MS and that they are directly caused by it. Like other symptoms, they can come and go and may be made worse by fatigue, infections or stress. People with these problems can get more muddled and confused in their thinking when tired. A few people with MS become severely disabled intellectually and are unable to cope with even simple tasks. This occurs mainly in those who also become severely disabled by physical problems, although not always so.

People with MS can appear irritable and over-sensitive at times. Relatives, in particular, can feel hurt and unjustly criticised. They may say that a person with MS has become selfish and is no longer able to see other peoples' problems. It may also be very hard for relatives to cope with the serious depression that can afflict people with MS; at these times both they and their relatives may need counselling and support.

These direct psychological symptoms are due to MS itself, but they may also be combined with the emotional upset that affects everyone when a family is trying to adapt to living with the disease. Once the symptoms associated with MS are recognised for what they are, then positive action can be taken to overcome them; for instance, someone who has a problem remembering things will find it useful to keep a note pad close at hand.

Recognising that these difficulties are due to MS can relieve a lot of guilt and frustration, and will help people to accept their illness more easily. But often there will be resistance by some of the people involved to the idea that mental symptoms can occur. This is entirely understandable; these particular symptoms are embarrassing and, certainly, they are some of the most frightening and the most upsetting in the whole disease.

I remember that when I first developed MS, I asked my neurologist whether mental symptoms might occur. He could not look at me and instead, looking sideways, said, 'Nonsense, nothing happens mentally at all; you'll be perfectly normal and don't worry about it.' He could not cope with the possibility of discussing these symptoms with me and I knew at the time he was not telling the strict truth, although for the best of reasons as far as he was concerned. Certainly in my case, the development of intellectual symptoms has been one of my great fears. I have now gone about twenty years with MS and am still able to cope with my work and live a normal life, and I hope that this will encourage many other people who are in the same position as I am. It should be stressed that many people with the disease will never experience these direct psychological symptoms and their disability will be confined to physical functions alone.

6   Coming to Terms with MS

When we discover that we have MS it usually comes as a great shock. This is to be expected; if it did not upset us we would be unusual indeed. It is normal and natural for us to be emotionally disturbed on learning the diagnosis and it is likely that we shall continue to be shaken for a considerable time. How we react to MS is in some ways like the experience of bereavement, but instead of having lost a loved one through death, we have lost our good health through illness. We have in fact lost a part of ourselves which we loved very much and we must instead take on a different identity, as 'a person who has MS' or as 'a disabled person'. It is necessary to mourn our loss if we are to make a good adjustment in the end, and this process can not be avoided or rushed.

When we lose a loved one through death, it may take months, or even years, before we can accept our loss. This is also true for MS, but not quite so straightforward and clear cut. We lose our good health gradually and slowly and we can never be sure how final the loss will be. We might be restored to health completely, sometimes partially but perhaps not at all, and this insecurity is very hard to bear. We may hardly have become used to one new self-image when we must abandon it and take on a different one.

Grief
It is not surprising that we must go through a period of sadness and grief. This is usually mixed with feelings of anger, and we may deny both to ourselves and others that we have the disease at all. Like the bereaved, a person who has MS must come to terms with his or her condition and learn to value him- or herself again and to enjoy living. This will take

time, perhaps several years, but much less time for some people than for others.

It seems that we have to experience shock, anger and sadness over and over again before we can become inwardly strong enough to be open and realistic about our limitations. When this stage is reached we shall have begun to come to terms with MS. Some people will be able to start leading a life just as fulfilling as before; a life that may be given more meaning by the experience of illness and suffering. But for others, there often appears to be no meaning left in life.

There are no short cuts but, like Virgil in Dante's *Inferno*, we must understand the secret: that the only exit from Hell is at its very centre. We can emerge from fear and depression when we have first accepted these feelings and been able to express them to ourselves and others.

Relatives also experience similar feelings of grief when someone in the family develops MS. Coupled with their grief, they may have complicated feelings of guilt and frustration, as well as a desire to be strong and supportive. When the whole family is faced with these complex feelings, they may not be able to support each other. They may require help from someone outside the family for a while, perhaps for a long time.

The emotional strain associated with MS can cause even more suffering and pain than the physical effects of the disease. This is true both for the person who has MS and for those close to him or her. The psychological process of adjusting to new identities, new roles and a new lifestyle is often long and complicated. For many, however, there will be unexpected rewards and fulfilment. Life sometimes appears as a random and purposeless experience from which we are asked to create meaning. For those of us with MS, and for our relatives, this is our particular challenge.

Early Fears

The first symptoms of MS are often irritating and confusing, and sometimes seem unimportant at the time. One person will experience double vision occurring for a short while, while another person will have pins and needles in her feet or fingers when particularly tired or hot. Yet another might experience undue tiredness in the afternoons and need to sleep more often in the daytime than is usual. He might also notice that a foot drags, causing him to stumble occasionally, or to trip on rough objects. These symptoms will often cause little concern at first, unless a person is well versed in medical matters or is particularly anxious about his or her physical health.

It begins to be more frightening when someone who has experienced these particular symptoms gets them more persistently or gets a mixture of the symptoms. Perhaps she will have experienced blurred vision for a week or two, with some pain in one eye, and six months later she might notice that she is dragging a foot. It is at this time that people usually go and see their doctor. It can be very alarming when we are first given a full examination and referred to a consultant neurologist. It is then that suspicion of something serious first appears not only to the people with the symptoms, but to those close to them. Investigations by the consultant neurologist in hospital or in the out-patient department may lead to increasing fears, especially if suspicions and anxieties are not shared and expressed. Many who eventually turn out to have MS are convinced that they have got a brain tumour and that no one will tell them the truth. Others suspect that they may be going mad, and that sooner or later they will be admitted to a psychiatric hospital.

Unfortunately, because the early symptoms of MS sometimes appear to the GP as symptoms of anxiety or depression, many patients are prescribed tranquillisers or other similar drugs at this time. They feel that they are being labelled as 'hypochondriacs', 'neurotics' or 'hysterics'. Some people are even referred to a psychiatrist. It is no wonder that they eventually become very anxious and depressed! I have come across a few people who have even been admitted to a psychiatric hospital before the diagnosis of MS has been made.

Relatives may also think that a person who has the early symptoms of MS is over-reacting and exaggerating in order to get attention. Both the person with MS and her relatives can feel misunderstood, hurt and very isolated at this time.

MS is not an easy diagnosis to make and, as I have explained in Chapter 4, it may be necessary to have a variety of investigations over quite a long period of time before the diagnosis can be made for certain. Many of us are quite shocked to learn that we have MS, but at the same time many people also feel relieved, especially if they had been fearing something worse. This relief can be short-lived, for it will not be long before the full impact of the disease sinks in. Initially there may also be disbelief; it may be very hard to accept that anything serious is wrong and some people go out of their way to find other explanations and even to consult other doctors.

Denial

Often, encouraged by their relatives, people will resort to all sorts of quack diets and treatments in order to try and find a cure for MS. This can be their way of refusing to accept reality, of pretending that MS is a curable disease, and it can lead them to spend vast quantities of money in order to buy useless treatments that may even be dangerous. Frequently associated with this is a feeling of anger towards orthodox medicine and doctors, sometimes justified, but sometimes exaggerated and unreasonable. We need to discredit those whose news we would rather not hear.

Denial of the symptoms of the disease can take many forms. Often people will not be able to admit to themselves that they have MS and it can take even longer before they can tell other people what their trouble really is. For this reason, families and employers are frequently excluded from knowing the true situation and may show little or no understanding.

Sharing Feelings

It is quite natural and normal to feel very angry about having MS, but it is important that this grief process, both the anger and the sadness, should be accepted and expressed. People need to cry, to be angry, to curse God and to ask, 'Why me?'

It is at this stage that doctors should consider the emotional needs of their patients as well as their physical requirements. Many people with MS look perfectly normal and the symptoms that they have been experiencing are quite invisible to others. But it is essential that they should be allowed to show their feelings, not only of anger, but also of sadness for the loss that has been experienced. This will require not only information, perhaps given by the GP in the surgery, but also opportunities to return to ask further questions; they need to receive care and time from a doctor as well as clinical efficiency and acumen. The counselling attitude necessary at this stage of the disease, when the diagnosis is being given to the patient, can be summed up in three words; time, attention and respect.

The Partner

Wives and husbands of people who have MS may also be grief-stricken and will need the same sort of help and support as their partners. In fact, it can be more difficult for them because they themselves do not have to suffer the disease. They can forget about it, perhaps, and deny the problem for longer.

They also face the guilt caused by the fact that it is their partner who has MS and not themselves, and they may try to compensate for this in all sorts of ways. It is made far more difficult for them if they have been given the diagnosis but told not to mention it. Keeping a secret like this from a partner is a very painful and difficult thing to do. Often, when the secret comes out, both partners will feel very angry, and this resentment will be directed not only at each other, but also at the doctor. This can cause a serious breakdown in the doctor-patient relationship, and even more difficulties in the marital relationship. (MS puts a great strain on marriages and families, as I shall explain in the next chapter.)

Loss of Self Respect

It is not just your good health that you have lost when you develop MS. Disability can lead not only to inconvenience, lack of mobility and frustration, but also to loss of work, loss of income and loss of status. A person who has been the breadwinner may find that he can no longer provide for his family and he may lose his self-respect and meaning in life. A mother who has always taken pride in running a home and bringing up her family may find herself cast aside while the house and family are run by others. This can be devastating, and can lead to a very serious depression if she is not helped to find an alternative role in the family and an alternative way of creating meaning in her life.

Further loss is caused by feeling dependent on others: by the inability to make decisions and carry them out on our own, and in having to rely on others as a child does on its parents. Work is an important part of life and loss of work, or a loss of future career prospects, can destroy a person's sense of fulfilment and belonging. It is a harrowing experience to find that our future expectations, perhaps of having a happy family life with several children, or a successful career, are dashed forever.

The sum total of loss – both these secondary losses and the loss of health that precedes them – leads to fundamental changes in how we see ourselves and in the relationships that we have with other people. These need to be understood and worked through before we can truly come to terms with MS.

Adjusting

People vary in the way they cope with disability. Some will be very disabled physically and yet will appear to cope well emotionally and to live a positive and rewarding life. Others will have very little by way of disability and yet find that they experience severe depression and a feeling that life has become meaningless. The reason for these differences is complicated and there are several factors involved.

Firstly, two people with the same symptom will each

experience it in a different way. Blurred vision and problems with reading will be more important to someone researching archives in the British Museum than to someone, a potter perhaps, who mainly uses his hands for his work. This is a rather simple way of looking at things, but we all react differently depending on how we see ourselves and our roles in life. Another factor is what sort of person we were before the illness struck; are you a happy-go-lucky individual who has coped easily with stress and succeeded in making adaptations when necessary? Or are you a fussy, anxious person who has never really felt able to cope when things went wrong? Again this is a simplification, but the personality of someone before she has MS is very important and will play a large part in determining how well she succeeds in adapting to the disease.

The stability of the family and the amount of support that they can give to the person with the disease is crucial, but so, too, is the attitude of the wider community and how much it is able to offer in the way of support and practical help to the whole family. If the person with MS has good employers who understand her special needs and requirements, this will help her to adjust at this point. A good local branch of the MS Society may also be an important factor. If there is a Welfare Officer or Support Group nearby it can be one way of sharing feelings about the disease and learning more about its consequences and ways of adjusting.

Critical Periods
There are many critical periods for people with MS as their dependency on other people increases. These are times when they will need particular understanding and counselling. I have already discussed the first of these – the time of diagnosis, when emotional help and support will be needed as well as information. It is the time when trust can be built up between doctors, nurses, social workers and the family with MS.

But there are other times when the person with MS will

need extra understanding. Perhaps the next one to occur, if the illness progresses, is when it becomes necessary to use some sort of walking aid. It can be very difficult to get used to a stick, as I know from my own experience, and can lead to feelings of selfconsciousness and embarrassment. Some people refuse to use these aids when they really need them and can be a nuisance to others. It seems to be a sign of getting worse, of increasing seriousness in the disease, and they may try to avoid facing this development.

The use of a wheelchair is a similar issue. Some people will do anything to avoid having to use wheelchairs because they see them as a sign of failure and uselessness. Others will be over-keen to use them when their disability is not severe. Or if incontinence occurs, it can be very embarrassing and another blow to self-respect. Many people, at this time, will not only need advice about where to obtain the relevant aids but also emotional support. When someone has to receive hospital treatment to go into some sort of residential care, even for a short time, a great deal of understanding and support will be required, not only by the person going into care, who will feel rejected and frightened, but also by the family and partner who may feel guilty and behave unreasonably and in a demanding fashion towards the professional carers.

In addition, coping with MS is made more complicated because many people also suffer from intellectual problems as a result of the disease. This can lead to difficulties with concentration and memory, as already discussed.

Coming to terms with MS is about finding the balance between, on the one hand, completely giving in to the disease and, on the other, completely denying it and refusing to accept it. I can think of several examples of both types of response when, instead of finding a balance, people have reacted in the extreme – perhaps all of us have a tendency to over-react one way or another before we find the middle-path way. I remember meeting a lady with very little disability who insisted on being pushed around in a wheelchair whenever possible. I found this particularly disturbing

DENIAL
Refusing to accept MS
Trying to live as though
  MS did not exist
Not adapting to changes
Blaming others for problems

OVER-ACCEPTANCE
Giving in to MS
Over-identifying with MS
Using MS as an excuse
Withdrawing from social
  contacts

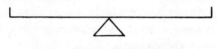

BALANCED ATTITUDE
Accepting limits, but not giving in to MS
Adapting to new ways of living, and to new roles
  at home and in the community
Living and contributing to the fullest extent possible
Creating new meanings and purposes in life

Fig 4. Coming to terms with MS.

because my own response has always been to the other
extreme. I have always been one of those people who
find it difficult to accept their illness and the idea of ever
going into a wheelchair horrifies me: I am sure that, if the
time should come, I would not be the easiest person to live
with for a while!

Maureen, whom I met a few years ago, was rather
different. While visiting her house, I noticed that she insisted
on washing all the dishes and cups after the family meal,
despite several breakages. I enquired into this, thinking that
perhaps this was an area she ought to avoid, due to her MS. I
discovered that she was uncompromising – this was her job
and she was going to continue doing it, despite all the broken
crockery! To make it worse, there were several teenagers in
the family, as well as her husband, who were very willing to
help. But this, for Maureen, made it all the more important
that she should continue her chaotic washing up; this was the
only way she felt she could find a role in the family. She was
denying her MS to a great extent, but over the years I hope
that she will accept her disability more readily and with more

grace. It was driving her family to distraction and not helping the relationships within it. This, unfortunately, is a frequent occurrence in MS.

On another occasion I met a middle-aged man who had an extremely good job as a top-ranking executive. He had been minimally affected by MS but he did suffer from fatigue, which he found hard to accept. This man, Michael, insisted on doing more than his colleagues, flying further in planes, getting bigger deals and so proving that he was 'normal'. Later Michael broke down into a depression and it was only when he had come through this that he was able to accept his limits.

Married couples vary in the way that they respond to the able-bodied community when one of them develops MS. Some choose to turn away from previous friends and acquaintances and make a new circle of friends from among the MS community in their local area. Other couples continue to interact socially with their able-bodied friends and neighbours and do not go out of their way to meet other people with the disease.

What suits one couple will not suit another; people with strong roots in their local community may feel accepted and well supported. But others may be more isolated, or feel that they have become 'different' or less acceptable. They may even have to move to a completely new locality for health reasons. These couples will particularly benefit from joining the local branch of the MS Society.

Acceptance
In any long term disease, we have to understand our limits and to find, through this understanding, what our new potential can be. If one door shuts, we may find another door opens. I have always found a quotation from the German poet, Goethe, to be of use to me whenever I am tempted to deny that I have MS and to try to do something really beyond my limits. Goethe wrote the following: 'It is in self-limitation that a master first shows himself.'

To me, this means that, if I am to be a master of living with MS, I must accept the particular limitations imposed on me by the disease that I have. Once I can accept these limitations, then I can go on to find some sort of meaning and satisfaction in life in spite of them, and perhaps even because of them. When we have come to terms with MS, and I do not believe that we ever fully do so, instead of asking, 'Why me?' we shall be able to ask, 'Why not me?' To answer this new question means that we must begin to accept our limits, realise our new potential and go on to create a new purpose for the rest of our lives.

7 Marriage under Stress

In England, during the so-called Dark Ages, there were no doctors or psychiatrists. But in those pagan times Anglo-Saxons did have healers and sorcerers who fulfilled a similar function. Healers worked with nature rather than against it, and they conceived of human beings as belonging to the natural world, not separate from it. Much of their knowledge and wisdom has been lost, but some of their old ideas remain. One of these is their view of the Universe as being like a four-dimensional cosmic cobweb. The natural world was seen as consisting of a system of inter-connecting invisible strands or fibres crossing time and space. If an event occurred in one part of the web, the vibrations would be felt in every other part. Put in a two-dimensional form, this is rather like the circle of ripples that is created when a stone is dropped into a pond.

This fantastic image, drawn from the natural world, illustrates an important truth, summed up in John Donne's famous words, 'No man is an island'. MS, like every other happening in the natural world, takes place in the universal cobweb of life. The strongest vibrations will be felt by those closest to the person who has the disease; but the effects of MS radiate beyond the immediate family and will make an impression and demand a response from friends, workmates and the community at large. Vibrations coming from the many people who have MS and from their families will, in turn, be felt throughout society, and eventually in the international community.

I have already described the changes that happen to the individual who has MS and how he or she must come to terms with a new identity and grieve for the loss of what might have been. I shall also explore the implications that MS can have for society and how the able-bodied respond to people with MS and their various disabilities and limitations. But in this chapter I intend to focus on that part of the 'cobweb' where the vibrations of MS are at their strongest: marriage and the family.

MS is not a disease that affects individual people in isolation. When one person in the family has MS, then the whole family 'has MS' as well. There will need to be changes in the relationships between the family members if the family as a whole is to adapt positively to the disease. This can mean fear, sadness and anger, not just for the person who has MS, but for all the members of the family in varying degrees.

'Whose MS?' – a dramatic sketch

Setting: our home on a Monday morning, just after the children have gone to school.

Cast: Sandy (myself, who has MS)
      Penny (my wife)

SANDY: What are you going to do today? I shall have to be late back this evening, so we may have to have tea later than usual.

PENNY: I shall be here all day and I have more than enough to get on with; there are so many little jobs that I really do not know where to start. It all just keeps piling up and no one seems to help.

SANDY: (*Angry, and feeling somewhat got at*) Well, I do try to do what I can, but as you should know by now, I have had MS for twenty years, and I get tired very quickly, especially when I have to work about the house, with all that bending and exercise. I can't help it – I did not ask for a virus to get stuck in my brain and make me feel ill all the time! I wish I felt well like you – I envy you and the girls for all your energy; I wish I felt fit and could take the dogs for a walk every day and feed the chickens. But I do not feel fit - I reckon I don't do too badly, considering . . .

PENNY: For goodness sake, stop going on, it just does not help me! I have got to put up with you and your MS as well. And I do not have any excuse to rest and leave jobs to anyone else. It is very trying, very depressing and I often feel unsupported. At least try to understand how *I* feel, sometimes. Are you surprised that I get angry and resentful?

SANDY: OK. You have made your point. MS is yours as well as mine. It is difficult for me to know how you feel when I get sorry for myself and angry because I cannot help my weaknesses. Thank you for letting me me know how things are from your point of view.

PENNY: It always helps when we are honest with each other.

THE END

Can I ever know how she feels? Do any of us who have MS know what it is like to be married to someone who has this disease? No, we cannot know. It is their experience, something that only our wives and husbands can share and understand. But we can at least acknowledge that they suffer, too. They are handicapped and disabled by MS in a different way but, like us, *they* have to mourn their loss and express their understandable anger and resentment.

Marriage

Marriage is difficult enough at the best of times; effort and attention are required by both parties if the relationship is to survive, let alone grow. When extra stress is added, such as an illness or a disability, then any cracks in the structure of the marriage may widen and eventually there can be a total collapse. The marriage breakdown rate is particularly high when one partner has MS, and this should not really surprise us. Perhaps more surprising is the fact that, despite the stresses and strains of MS, so many relationships not only survive, but grow in strength.

MS is often blamed for the breakdown of a marriage, but is this really fair? Certainly it is a factor in marriage break-downs, but what was the relationship like to begin with? It is all very well being able to live with someone when everything goes well and there are no problems, but that is a fairy-tale world, not the real world in which real people have to live. Every marriage will be subjected to stress from one source or another. Perhaps it is illness or financial loss, perhaps it is the presence of a mentally handicapped child or an illicit love affair. MS, like other hurdles, can be unfairly scapegoated as the cause of marriage breakdowns when in fact the marriage was weak in the first place.

Nevertheless, there is no doubt that MS is a particularly unkind and destructive influence, and many marriages do not survive its impact. Despite this, and sometimes after much emotional pain, a couple will be able to turn the experience upside down and may learn to understand each other better and learn to accept each other's limitations in a more positive way. I wish this occurred more often, but certainly I have met several couples to whom this has happened.

The Stress of MS
I do not want to minimise the destructive power that MS has on relationships, and it is important to understand what can happen when things go wrong. Marriage and family life are not what they used to be; the 'extended families' of the past could absorb illness and provide support in a way that the small 'nuclear family' of today cannot. Instead the caring and support that used to be provided by those numerous uncles, aunts, cousins and grandparents now often has to come from the local authority, or even from the state. It is perhaps too much to expect a working wife or husband to be able to cope with a chronically sick partner and a young family all at the same time! Without help something will have to go – maybe the marriage; maybe the job; maybe the children.

Both partners need to mourn their loss and, if they become

depressed at the same time, it will not be easy for them to help each other. Instead, they may feel unsupported and resentful towards one another. Wives and husbands may feel uncertain about how far to push the partner who has MS, and may not be able to distinguish between difficult behaviour which is really due to MS, and behaviour which is due to normal selfishness or bloody mindedness!

A caring partner may feel overwhelmed and exhausted by the constant demands made on her by someone who has MS, and may feel trapped in the relationship. She may find it impossible to cope with her partner's depression, irritability and self-pity and may desperately need someone to care for her, too, sometimes, and to understand her needs. However, some people will feel emotionally 'threatened' by help from those outside the immediate family and may resent the invasion of privacy and the implication that they cannot cope on their own. Well-meaning helpers should be careful not to make a caring wife or husband feel incompetent or redundant.

Anger
Sometimes it is difficult for the caring relative to be angry with a partner who has MS. This can be because she feels guilty, and because she does not want to hurt someone who is already vulnerable and dependent, through no fault of his own. On the other hand, the person who has MS may also feel angry. He may have lost his role as 'the bread winner' in a family and may resent being dependent and having to rely on his partner. He, too, may feel unable to express his anger, in case he is rejected by the person who has control over him. This anger can gradually build up until it either explodes or turns into severe depression.

When both partners are unable to acknowledge their natural aggression and resentment, then their relationship is bound to suffer. The anger may come out indirectly and appear as rejection or as over-protection by the caring partner; they each need to distance themselves from the person who causes so much trouble. Or the person with MS may become manipulative and begin to play on the partner's feelings of guilt. Sometimes a person with MS will gain a great deal from being treated as an invalid and will exaggerate his symptoms in order to get attention and pity. However, this can increase the distance between the partners and cause even more anger and resentment from the person who has to care for him.

One couple in particular comes to my mind as an example of this unacknowledged anger and its destructive effects. In their case the wife, who was previously a strong, independent woman, developed MS and the husband had to look after her. One of his jobs was to push her wheelchair and to take her wherever she wanted to go. The wife complained that he used to leave her for ages in the bathroom and that he did not respond, even to prolonged and frantic shouting! When I asked him why this was, he just looked at the floor and then quietly said that he had noticed that he had begun to be a little bit deaf. He added that he had not heard his wife shouting because he had been out in the garden.

It was clear to me that being 'deaf' and 'out in the garden' were the only ways that this man could get back at his demanding wife without overtly opposing her and showing anger. In this case neither partner was fully able to admit his or her anger towards the other, despite the dramatic change in their circumstances and the woman's increasing dependence on her not very willing husband. They had originally come to see me because of a sexual problem. What emerged from our session was not so much sexual problems, as unexpressed anger on both sides, which was making intimacy and sex an impossibility.

It seems that many people are frightened of admitting or expressing their anger; it is almost as if there is a taboo against anger, rather like there used to be about sex. Sex is certainly discussed quite openly these days; the popular press dwells on every aspect of sexuality at length and at regular intervals! On the other hand, 'Oh no! I am not angry' is a regular refrain, despite evident frustration, resentment and provocation.

Why do we deny our anger? Is it fear? Has anger become socially unacceptable? Is it a sign of weakness in our society? It is all these things and more. We live in a violent world and perhaps it is hard for people to differentiate between real violence and destructive aggression and natural and normal anger or assertiveness. This is a pity, because the bottling up of anger can eventually lead to depression, to hate in a relationship, or to an eventual violent reaction.

> I was angry with my friend;
> I told my wrath, my wrath did end.
> I was angry with my foe:
> I told it not, my wrath did grow.
>
> William Blake

The very thing that people hope to avoid – violence – can become more likely to happen when they are unable or unwilling to admit their angry feelings towards one another. The opposite is also true. Once we can openly say to someone, 'I am angry with you,' this can lead to deeper honesty and love in a relationship. But saying that we are angry is not the same as saying, 'You make me angry,' or, 'It is your fault that I am angry'. These responses are destructive and are made by a person who is not taking responsibility for himself. He is trying to force another person to feel responsible or guilty for his own feelings.

We all need to realise that anger is not necessarily bad or destructive. It is a natural reaction to frustration or misunderstanding, and admitting this to ourselves is often the best way of putting things right. By doing this we can help other people to take responsibility for their feelings and behaviour, and some sort of adult solution will be found to the problems. Usually there are misunderstandings and mistakes on both sides, and each person needs to give as well as to take in a relationship.

By treating anger in this way we are behaving as adults. I am not suggesting that we go to extremes and shout and scream as soon as we feel under strain! This would be a childish response; we have to be mature enough to choose the right time and the right way to express our anger, not any old place at any old time. Self-control is just as important as freedom of expression, and they must go together if we are to get the balance right. Perhaps I can compare it to fire which can be a creative and helpful aid to mankind; but if it gets out of control it can be destructive and disastrous. Fire and anger are similar; they are not in themselves good or bad, it all depends on what we do with them.

Misunderstandings

I have spent some time discussing the importance of anger in relationships because it is fundamental to many of the difficulties that occur between people when someone has MS. Anger can lead to complete rejection of another person. She no longer seems to be 'the same person that I married'. The implication is that the person with MS has changed on purpose and is no longer prepared to play her part in the relationship as she used to before she was ill.

The partner may feel let down, rejected, and treated badly; he may consider that the person who has MS is selfish and not prepared to see things from any point of view other than her own. This sort of misunderstanding might occur less often if people with MS and their partners had more realistic expectations of one another. Very often the effects of fatigue are poorly understood and can lead to resentment on the part of partners because they think that their wife or husband is 'not trying' or 'pulling a fast one'.

I have already explored these problems in Chapter 5, together with the other difficulties that can occur if someone with MS has psychological impairment caused directly by the MS disease process. It is unfortunately true that there are occasions when people with MS are selfish and over-demanding, and their unreasonable behaviour may be taken personally by their partners. It is hard to understand that a person with MS has lost his ability to see things from another point of view as a result of MS and not through any fault of his own. When marriages break down for these reasons the guilt and frustration experienced by the partners can be great, and they may genuinely not be able to understand or to cope with what has been happening. This situation is tragic for the whole family. These difficulties need to be understand for what they are – symptoms of MS, and not 'bloody mindedness' – so that information and support can be offered to the relatives at an early stage.

Of course, not all difficult behaviour should be blamed on the disease – people with MS *can* be 'bloody minded' at times like everyone else! Relatives may find it difficult to judge what are the true mental effects of the disease and which are emotional reactions to having MS, such as depression, anger or guilt.

Over-Protection

A caring relative will sometimes respond in an over-protective way and the couple may then become particularly close and exclude others from their life. But there is a price to pay for this way of trying to cope. The couple can lose their adult type of relationship and may develop a 'parent/child' one instead. This is an understandable way of responding but it can lead to resentment and frustration in the relationship and to suspicion of outsiders or withdrawal from the outside world.

I have seen this happening on a number of occasions and it is a difficult pattern to alter, even when it is seen to be destructive to both partners. It is in fact a way of dealing with anxiety, guilt and a fear of rejection by the other person concerned. It allows the couple to stay together; they continue to be needed by each other but for reasons different from before. They may consequently avoid facing up to the changes and demands of a more equal and adult relationship.

I once read a bizarre story about a man and a woman who married but had no children. She began to 'mother' her husband who quickly fell into a dependent role, taking less and less responsibility for himself as time went on. The man grew smaller, becoming shorter and younger until it was not long before he turned into a little boy. Eventually he became a baby and his wife/mother began to push him around in a pram. Finally he just shrivelled up and disappeared altogether!

This horrible story has a little truth in it, for it illustrates what can happen to people who have an unequal relationship, when one person is over-dependent on the other. They can lose their identity as individual adults and may instead take the parts of child and parent until there is nothing left between them except stereotyped roles.

Parents

A similar dilemma can develop in families when one or both parents of a person who has MS begin to treat their grown-up son or daughter as a child again. Perhaps they feel guilty in some way about what has happened and their help may be needed, but the end result can be destructive if they go too far. Sometimes parents of a person with MS blame their son- or daughter-in-law for not caring for their 'child' properly and may even suggest that the partner is the cause of the illness!

I have known this sort of parental interference be a factor in the break-up of marriages and the tragedy is that the parents have usually convinced themselves that they are doing the right thing. This is an extreme example, but MS families seem to have more than their fair share of in-law problems. Couples may find that, instead of receiving support they are the recipients of unhelpful and rejecting responses from one or other set of parents, and they may not know how to react.

It must be difficult for parents to accept that one of their 'children' has developed an incurable disease and I can well understand that many wish to deny the truth, or to find some factor or person to blame. Several couples have told me that they wished that they had never mentioned MS to their parents or in-laws because it had made matters so much worse. It is clear that, in some circumstances, parents and in-laws could usefully be offered information and counselling from a professional; they, too, may need to work through guilt feelings and anger about what has happened.

If a son or daughter who has MS is single, then the parents will usually be more directly involved from the outset. There is again the danger that they will react by becoming more parental, by taking over responsibility for the person affected who may be treated more and more like a child. The person concerned may have grown up, become independent and left home when all of a sudden she finds herself back to 'square one'. She will often feel depressed at having lost her hard-won independence and freedom and she can feel angry and resentful, in particular towards her parents.

The parents, in their turn, may not be pleased that they are lumbered with a 'dependent child' just when they had thought that they would have more time for themselves; they, too, can feel resentful and consequently might also feel guilty. It is at this stage that a vicious circle can begin to develop. In situations like this it will often be useful to have advice and support from a neutral person. A social worker can help both in counselling the family, and in arranging accommodation for the person who has MS, in order that she can maintain her independence. If she cannot live on her own with MS, it may be best for her to be offered residential care rather than go back and live with her parents. Although some people may feel this is avoiding their responsibilities, it will make it easier for the person who has MS, and for her parents, to retain their previous adult relationship. It will also help them avoid the many difficulties that can so easily occur when a sick or disabled person is looked after by her parents.

Every situation is different, and there will be occasions when it will be considered best all round for a person with MS to be looked after by her parents. In these cases it is essential that adequate support is provided and that both caring parents and dependent persons with MS are given breaks from one another as often as they need them.

Helpful Families

It may seem that I have criticised parents too much and I need to add that parents, in-laws and family members usually play a valuable and constructive part in supporting people who have MS, as well as their partners. They can share in some of the practical care that may have to take place and they can often relieve the pressure on an exhausted partner.

I have been especially fortunate in having a supportive wife, despite the fact that I am not always the easiest person to live with! In the past I received much help and understanding from my father when he was alive, and my mother has always been available and willing to assist whenever I needed her. Penny's parents live farther away but, despite this, they have consistently played an important role in coming to our aid when needed, and in giving us breaks and help with our children and animals. They are also actively involved in the work of the MS Society in their own area. In addition, I am lucky in having my brothers and sisters, together with their families, nearby; all of them help out at times as a natural part of family life.

It is easy to be smug, and I am conscious that, without the continuing support of my family and friends, my life could have been very different, and I doubt whether I could have been so active in the MS movement. It is impossible to over-estimate the part that others play in enabling us to cope with illness and disability: I hope that I shall never take my family and friends for granted, and that the families and friends of others reading this will realise their importance and worth.

As far as marriage itself is concerned, I should like to give the final words of this chapter to the Lebanese poet, Khalil Gibran,

> And stand together yet not too near together:
> For the pillars of the temple stand apart,
> And the oak tree and the cypress grow not
>   in each other's shadow.

8 Sex, Pregnancy and Children

Affection and physical contact are basic needs for everyone; we only have to look at the way that babies and children are brought up, or the way that young animals are fondled, licked and nuzzled, to realize how important it is to have physical contact from an early age. But adults also need to be touched, caressed and hugged to remain healthy individuals. An American psychologist has said that every person needs at least four big hugs a day, but I wonder how many people get their fair share?

It has been shown that an important factor in prolonging someone's life after a heart attack is whether there are pets at home. The simple habit of stroking a warm, furry animal can bring down the blood pressure and cause a deep feeling of relaxation. Research carried out in an Intensive Care Unit found that those people whose hands were held, even though they appeared to be unconscious, survived more frequently than those who were left entirely isolated without any human contact.

There are many cultural attitudes influencing the way that we respond to one another. I remember that, when I visited Vienna, I was very embarrassed when I was hugged and kissed on both cheeks by the big, strong, hairy husband of a distant relative of mine. It was difficult to explain to the amazed on-lookers, many of whom were staying in the same hotel with me and attending an MS Society conference! The Viennese are certainly much better than the British at demonstrating physical affection and I am sure that we have a lot to learn from them.

Even within my British culture there are many differing

attitudes to touch, and I remember seeing a couple who came for help because one of them had MS. The wife, Melanie, complained that her husband, James, had not been paying enough attention to her sexually since their marriage. James had MS, but this did not seem to be the main problem. Melanie said that all had been well between them sexually before their marriage, but since that time James had just been 'turning his back on her in bed at night, and going to sleep'.

It turned out that their backgrounds were very different. Melanie had been the youngest girl in the family and she had spent much of her life being praised, complimented and told how pretty she was; she had frequently been cuddled and dandled on her father's knee as a child. James's experience of physical contact was different: for him, physical contact was associated with the many times that his father had 'given him the strap' for bad behaviour. The more that Melanie pestered James (as he saw it), the more negative he became, and a vicious circle had developed. It eventually became clear that it was not just sexual intercourse that Melanie really wanted, although this was quite possible physically for James; she just needed an occasional cuddle and reassurance about her femininity.

It is easy to touch people who have been bereaved, to hold their hands or to put your arms round them; but touching someone who is suffering from depression is much more difficult. They seem to be unresponsive, undeserving and generally self-pitying. Touching disabled people can often be difficult, too; disability can cause feelings of revulsion and fear. Disabled people can also feel a sense of self-revulsion and think that they are unattractive to others or undeserving of a physical or sexual relationship. This poor self-image often leads to a complete withdrawal from social or sexual relationships, or occasionally to the opposite: a craving for reassurance and an attempt to over-compensate by making demands that can be unacceptable to others.

SEXUAL PROBLEMS

Many people who have MS experience sexual problems of one sort or another during the course of their illness. Sexual problems are common, anyway, in the general population, and when someone with MS complains that his sex life is not satisfactory, the cause could be any one of several different factors, or a mixture of them.

MS often has a direct effect on sexual functioning, due to neurological damage associated with the demyelination of certain parts of the spinal cord. Men can experience difficulty in getting or maintaining an erection, and at times complete impotence can occur. They may also notice changes in the timing or the nature of ejaculation, or of orgasm. Sensory problems, or even pain, can be experienced in the genital region, and ejaculation or orgasm may become painful rather than pleasurable. They may also experience the more general symptoms of weakness, fatigue or muscle spasm, and any of these can make sexual contact more difficult.

Equivalent difficulties can occur in women who may experience lack of vaginal lubrication and the absence of the clitoral engorgement which precedes orgasm. Women, too, can develop numbness or painful sensations in the genital region and, as in men, sex can be unpleasant on account of weakness, fatigue or muscle spasms.

Sexual symptoms vary from person to person and individuals may find that, like any other symptom of MS, they wax and wane in association with relapses, remissions and fatigue. Nevertheless, many people have long-lasting sexual difficulties which can cause anxiety, a negative self-image and depression, and these in turn will frequently be the cause of increased stress on relationships with sexual partners.

Psychological Influences

In the population as a whole, psychological problems commonly lead to sexual difficulties. When I was a medical student I was taught that 'the commonest cause of impotence is impotence'. This means that once someone has experienced impotence or a sexual 'failure', his anxiety will be much greater next time he tries. The result is an escalation of difficulties because the anxiety or the fear of failure will make it even more likely that impotence will occur again – and so on.

Sometimes MS couples avoid sexual intercourse in order to minimise feelings of failure and frustration, and this can lead to resentment if the situation is not talked over openly, without the partners blaming each other for what has happened. Sexual drive and habits vary considerably among all sections of the population; there is no 'right way' of relating to someone sexually any more than there is a right time, or a right frequency of sexual intercourse. Every couple will go through phases, and problems should only become a source of irritation if two people cannot communicate with each other and do not attempt to understand each other's needs.

Very often the sexual drive, or the libido, of one partner will exceed that of the other, due perhaps to illness, fatigue or other factors. In these cases masturbation (sexual self-stimulation) can provide an outlet and relieve sexual frustrations when a partner finds that the other does not wish to take part at that time. In the past, masturbation was regarded as wicked and was thought to be the cause of many diseases. Now this is known to be quite untrue, and many hold the alternative view: that masturbation can actually help people to stay healthy by relieving normal tensions. Masturbation was even thought to be the cause of MS at one stage: there was a theory that the over-frequent production of semen could lead to loss of fluid from the brain via the spinal cord!

I remember talking to a woman whose husband had MS, about their sexual problems. Her attitude was sensible and refreshing, and she commented. 'Whether someone is disabled or not, does not really matter. Some people will always have sexual problems, whilst others will adjust whatever happens.'

Relationships

It is easy to scapegoat MS as the cause of all marital or sexual problems, even though the relationship might not have been strong before the onset of the disease. I have already described the effects of unexpressed anger between partners, and how it may mean that intimacy or sexual relations become an impossibility. The general nature of the relationship that two people have with one another is crucial to how they cope when things go wrong. When one or both partners have a rigid view of sex and feel guilty if they do something that they regard as 'wrong' or 'unorthodox', then they are less likely to adjust or feel able to experiment. Some people believe that the only right way to have sex is conventional genital sexual intercourse and that anything else is 'dirty', 'perverted' or 'like animals'.

There is, however, increasing evidence to suggest that this view of intercourse is over-rated. Studies have shown that for many women, possibly even for the majority, genital intercourse is not necessarily the best way of achieving physical or psychological satisfaction. Apparently many women find that they can be aroused and obtain an orgasm more effectively through manual (using the hands) or oral (using the mouth) stimulation. If this is true, the penis has certainly been over-valued. This information may surprise men who identify strongly with that particular organ, but it could help those who have experienced impotence to feel less badly about it, and to realise that they might be able to give pleasure to their partner in other ways, and perhaps even more effectively than they did before.

Adapting

When sexual problems do occur, for either physical or psychological reasons, there are various ways of improving the situation. If, for instance, vaginal lubrication is lacking, this can easily be remedied by using KY Jelly which can be obtained over the counter at most chemists or drug stores. Since it is used for a wide variety of medical problems, there is no need to feel embarrassed. Some people find that sexual aids such as a penile prosthesis (false penis) or a 'vibrator' will enable them to achieve a happier and more fulfilled sexual relationship. There is nothing 'wrong' with using such aids if they are acceptable to both partners.

Above all, it is necessary to change attitudes when these are narrow or unimaginative. Sexual experimentation can lead to new ways of giving one another pleasure and there is some evidence that people who are disabled often enjoy a sex life with their partners that is more varied and imaginative than that of many able-bodied people. Those who are disabled may *have* to make adjustments and to experiment!

Despite the fact that alternative sexual techniques are available, some people feel guilty about this and may find it impossible to experiment, for instance with manual or oral sexual stimulation. What will suit one couple will not suit another, but there is no reason to give up in despair. Information and counselling can help couples to make the best of their sexual potential and there is no longer any excuse for a doctor to say, 'It is all part of your MS – you will have to learn to live with it.'

A sexual relationship of one sort or another is always possible; even women with catheters can have sexual intercourse, provided that care is taken to avoid bladder infections and that the catheter is positioned properly. Some people with MS worry that they will lose control of their bladder or bowels during sexual activity, but this can be avoided by going to the lavatory before sexual activity commences. In men, catheterisation gives rise to obvious sexual problems. But it may not be necessary to keep the catheter in all the time – this should be discussed with a sympathetic doctor. In particular, if the main problem is night-time incontinence, then a useful alternative is to wear a penile sheath leading to a urine bag. This is preferable for both medical and personal reasons.

Sometimes it is necessary to find the most comfortable position when sexual activity is complicated by weakness,

spasm or fatigue. Couples should be encouraged to experiment as much as possible, without always taking themselves
too seriously. When anxiety and fear of failure are making
matters worse, it may be useful for partners to practise
caressing and stroking one another, without attempting
genital stimulation or intercourse, for a specific period of
time. This sometimes diminishes anxiety by taking the
pressure off having to 'perform'. It can actually lead to a more
successful sexual relationship because the couple are able
simply to enjoy their intimacy and love-making, without
unrealistic expectations getting in the way.

It is important to maintain opportunities for intimacy.
Single beds have many advantages, but they have obvious
disadvantages as well! And moving the bed downstairs may
make privacy impossible. It is quite simple to install a chair-
lift on the stairs of most houses, and this enables the disabled
partner to use the whole house.

Help from Others

If couples cannot find a solution to their particular
problem, a family doctor will often be able to help or to
recommend a specialised therapist or clinic. There is also a
charity called Sexual and Personal Relationships of the
Disabled (SPOD) which exists in Britain especially to cater
for the needs of disabled people with relationship problems.
They produce useful literature and they also organise talks
and study days. In addition, they may suggest other ways of
getting help. The MS Society is also able to offer help, and I
recommend the Canadian MS Society booklet *Sexuality and
MS*, which is available from the MS Society or from SPOD.

Living away from Home

When a person who has MS is living away from home in
residential care or in a hospital, it may be difficult, through
lack of privacy, to maintain any sort of sexual relationship.
However, the staff at such centres are these days becoming
more sensitive to such needs, and sometimes a partner will be

allowed to stay in the resident's room. Unfortunately, this does not happen everywhere, and often a seriously disabled person will not be expected to want or to need sexual contact. Attitudes of this sort can be destructive to marital or other close relationships, and I shall examine the problem in more depth when considering residential care and self-respect.

When partners are separated, it is easy for jealousy to arise. Someone who is unable to have a normal sexual relationship for any reason may suspect that his or her partner is going elsewhere for sexual satisfaction. This worry is understandable and frequently occurs when someone with MS has to live away from home. Jealous feelings need to be talked about openly and attempts should be made to ensure that the sexual relationship between the couple can continue even though one of them is away from home.

Another sort of jealousy involves the partner of someone who has MS. I heard the following story from an elderly lady. Her husband, severely disabled with MS, lived in a Cheshire Home about thirty miles away. She visited him weekly and was pleased that he seemed to be quite happy there. But she disliked the fact that young women helped at the Home, and that they had intimate contact with her husband because they helped to nurse and wash him. She was quite jealous of these girls and I remember being surprised that a woman with an extremely disabled husband should feel this way. I had not until that time realised how a partner might feel in this situation, and it seemed sad to me that she felt so excluded and jealous. Staff at Cheshire Homes and similar residential establishments need to be aware that these sorts of feelings are experienced by partners as well as residents, and both partners need to be offered counselling and emotional support.

Nurse or Lover
Sometimes a partner or close relative has to nurse a sick husband or wife, and this can have a stressful effect on their marriage if the partner becomes a 'nurse' rather than a

'lover'. Having to do all the nursing and washing for a very disabled partner can be a sexual turn-off and may leave no room for intimate caressing or love-making. Although community nurses and remedial therapists often train and encourage partners to carry out nursing or other therapies, and partners are frequently keen to help, this can mean that the marriage will lose some of its magic; instead of a lover, the disabled partner can be left with an exhausted, 'turned off' and resentful 'nurse'.

Relatives and partners should not feel obliged to do these jobs unless they particularly want to (which some of them do), and community nurses and therapists should be aware of the problems. In some cases it would be better for nursing and medical procedures to be carried out by someone other than the relative. This would mean that the caring relative could continue purely in the role of wife or husband. In some situations this might save a marriage and allow it to become happier and more fulfilling. But in other circumstances, relatives will regard nursing their partner as their own responsibility and will not wish other people to become involved in such intimate tasks. In these cases they should be given every opportunity to care for their disabled partner in whatever way that they feel is appropriate, There are no 'rights or wrongs' in such matters. Some people are more squeamish than others when it comes to bodily functions, and not everyone is a natural nurse. What one person can cope with easily may really upset another, through no fault of his or her own. People are constitutionally different in this respect, and it is wrong to criticise others just because they happen to be different.

Sexual problems can lie at the root of marital difficulties, jealousy, and resentment, and it is essential to do something about them at the earliest opportunity. Usually this will involve talking things over with the partner honestly and without anger. It is especially helpful to share feelings about likes, dislikes and expectations and it is important for each partner to tell the other what he or she would like to be

different. As is so often the case in MS, they may not be able to
alter the physical symptoms or the problem itself, but two
people who care for each other may often be able to find a
different but acceptable way of meeting each other's needs.

PREGNANCY
A difficult decision faced by younger people who have MS,
and by their wives and husbands, is whether to begin a family
or whether to have further children. It is common for women
to associate the onset of their MS with the birth of a child and
in the past some doctors used to advise against having
children at all if MS was diagnosed. But does pregnancy
actually make MS worse? Or can pregnancy be the cause of
the condition? It is certainly true that MS is commonly first
noticed after a baby is born, but this could be because having
babies and developing MS both usually occur in the age
group of young adults. In other words, the association might
be purely coincidental. Evidence from studies on the long-
term effects of MS in women who have had a pregnancy and
in women who have not, shows that pregnancies make no
difference to the eventual degree of disability in the long
term. In fact, many women who have MS feel better during a
pregnancy, when many symptoms remit or become less
severe. On the other hand, relapses often take place in the few
months after the birth of a baby.

Making Decisions
So, should a woman diagnosed as having MS start a family?
This is a question that only the person concerned can answer,
preferably after discussion with her partner. Although
pregnancy does not influence the course of MS, the stress of
looking after babies and small children has to be considered,
not to mention the strain of bringing up older children and
teenagers. At the onset of the disease, it is difficult to say how
disabled a person will become. Once five years have passed a
doctor may often be in a position to advise on the possible
outcome. In general, if someone is already quite disabled

after five years, then the long-term outlook may not be so good as in the case of someone who is relatively well after five years. But this is a general rule, and individuals may very well prove to be exceptions. If they are young, it may be best for a couple to wait a few years before making any firm decision, but this advice might not be appropriate with older couples who have less time. Women with MS are just as fertile as other women, and MS does not in any way influence their chance of becoming pregnant.

Another cause of concern to couples is whether their children might possibly inherit MS. As I explained in Chapter 1, there is a slightly increased risk of developing MS among close relatives, including the children of someone who has the disease, but the risk is very small indeed, and MS is not an inherited disease. The couple may need to discuss this slight risk with a doctor or with a counsellor, but in the end they will have to make their own decision. Many decide to have children and nearly all of these grow up to be quite healthy.

Contraception
If a couple decide not to have children or to have no further children, then they must consider the best method of contraception. Vasectomy in men or sterilisation in women are not associated with any special extra risk for people with MS, and there is no evidence that taking the contraceptive pill will influence the course of MS one way or the other. If either of these methods is chosen, the doctor will take MS into consideration and should assess his patient with special care, including regular check-ups for those on the pill. The intra uterine device (IUD) may not be a sensible choice for some women, especially if they are prone to strong leg spasms, or when they lack sensation in their abdominal or pelvic regions.

Alternatives
If a couple wish to have their own children but the man has problems with ejaculation or erection, then artificial

insemination (AI) can be considered; MS does not affect the fertility of sperm in a man. Alternatively, couples who cannot, or do not wish to have their own children might consider adopting, like any other couple. But both partners will need to have a medical examination and the presence of MS may be considered a negative factor. This is not always the case, and people with MS but only slight disability are sometimes given the benefit of the doubt, especially if the disease appears to be running a benign course. Obviously, it is necessary to make sure that both partners are capable of being good parents, since a child's future will be at stake.

When pregnancy, contraception and other issues of this nature are being considered, it is essential that couples seek advice from their family doctor and that they are able to ask questions and to make their decisions when they have obtained all the information they need. A person offering counselling in such situations, and in the case of sexual problems, will not only need listening skills but should have up-to-date and accurate information about MS itself. Such information is always available from the MS Society who are backed up by a panel of experts and scientists.

In our own case, Penny and I found that, after several years of marriage, she had not become pregnant. This was nothing to do with my own MS, since I was relatively little affected, but, like one in eight couples, we had to accept that we were infertile. Although disappointed, we still wanted to have children and we were both aware that there were many children who need parents. We applied and were accepted as foster parents. Clare and Sarah came to us when they were aged seven and five respectively, and they have now been with us for nearly five years. We made a decision to have two children rather than one, so that they could be company for each other. We also stipulated that we would like our children to be of school age, so as to minimise the strain and to allow for my MS and fatigue problems. We are now in the process of adopting our two girls. My MS has not so far been any great difficulty for either of us as parents, or for the children. We have come to accept the ups and downs of family life, and we also enjoy the rewards that children bring.

CHILDREN

Last winter one of my daughters took part in an audition for the local Christmas pantomime. She was successful and, being a natural young actress and dancer, she loves to take part in all such productions, given a half a chance! When she came home she told me that a friend's father was going to be in the pantomime. 'You are as funny as him,' she said, 'if you did not have MS you could have been in the pantomime like him.' She went on to tell me at length how she had explained to her friend why I was not at the audition. 'Because he cannot leap about the stage – he has a disease that makes him go slowly and he has to use a stick.'

It is an unfortunate fact that MS most commonly develops at the time when many people are getting married and bringing up their children. The impact of MS on family life and on the emotional development of children can be immense and I have come across several families in which the children have been under great pressure. For instance, I have known more than one occasion in which the stress was so great that it resulted in a teenage member of the family attempting suicide. I have also come across families in which one or more children have been received into the care of the local authority because they have been uncontrollable at home and the parent or parents were completely unable to look after them. In one case an eight year-old boy attempted to burn down the family home.

When someone in a family is disabled a great strain is, of course, placed on the fit partner, and I have already discussed what can happen in such relationships. This strain is much greater when there are also young children in the family who have to be cared for and disciplined. In such situations it is not surprising that the caring partner often finds she cannot cope, and this results in great distress for the children. On occasions, the fit partner will find the pressures so great that she walks out of the family, leaving the disabled person to bring up the children on his own. This is an extremely difficult task and, if there is insufficient support from family or friends, then the social work department may be able to help by 'sharing the caring'. Help can include providing a 'home help', adapting the house, or arranging for the children to be fostered for a while, in order to give the parent a break. In some circumstances the child may have to be admitted to a children's home; this will put further strain on family relationships and will result in increased stress for the child concerned.

Children at Home

I have described some of the more tragic difficulties that can occur when one person in a family has MS, but a great many problems experienced by children and families can be dealt with at home. It is amazing how well some families adapt and how successful parents can be in changing their roles and lifestyles in order to meet the needs of their children.

Parents can sometimes be unsure how much to tell small children about MS, and whether the whole subject should best be kept secret in order to avoid distressing them. It is difficult to find the right balance between the two extremes – of telling the children too much or else nothing at all. But children can be very sensitive to what is not said and often worry far more when parents have a secret, than if the facts are explained to them at a level they can understand.

Some children will think that their parent is very ill or about to die, and they may not be able to express their terrors openly for fear of upsetting their parents. This is disturbing not only for the child concerned, but also for the relationship that the child has with his or her parents. It may lead to serious behaviour difficulties, suicide attempts or problems at school, such as bullying other children or failing to cope with normal school work. It is better to bring worries out in the open and discuss them than to 'bottle them up'.

Children can sometimes be embarrassed when accompanying a disabled parent in a public place and may refuse to be seen with their mother or father in these circumstances. This can result in the parent feeling rejected and in turn becoming angry with the child, which only makes the problem worse. Some children who have a parent with MS can feel jealous of those who have healthy parents. A girl may miss the experience of going shopping with her mother, or a boy might be resentful and envious of other boys who are able to play football with their fathers.

Children can sometimes feel guilty because their mother or father has MS and may quite unreasonably blame themselves either for being the cause of the disease, or for being an extra burden on their parents. In extreme cases this, too, can lead to a teenager taking an overdose of tablets, or to other self-destructive gestures. Guilty feelings are obviously not helped by those mothers who associate the onset of their MS with the birth of their child in a futile attempt to find some reason for developing the disease!

In cases like this, it may be helpful for the whole family to be seen together at a Child and Family Guidance Centre. Social workers or psychiatrists at such a centre may offer assessment or therapy, with the aim of encouraging families to be more open about their anxiety and frustrations, and about their expectations of one another, so that the channels of communication between them can be improved.

Answering Questions
Family secrets usually cause more problems than they solve, so children need to be involved in understanding their parents' difficulties. Young children will usually ask questions if they are given the chance, and they will accept answers that explain the situation at their own level of understanding.

'Why does mummy have to use a stick?'

'Because her legs are wobbly and a stick helps her to walk better.'

'Why are mummy's legs wobbly?'

'Because she has had an illness which has made it difficult

for messages from her brain to get to her leg muscles. When she tries to make her legs work, they do not move properly and she gets wobbly. If she uses a stick this helps her to feel steadier and to walk better.'

'Shall I get this illness, too?'

This last question is a common worry for children, and it is important that they realise that MS is not a hereditary disease and that it is most unlikely that they will ever get it. It is also necessary to explain that the disease is not 'catching' (infectious or contagious).

The more honestly that children's questions are dealt with and answered, the more satisfied and secure they will feel. As time goes on there will be opportunities to explain MS to them little by little, making sure that they understand about fatigue and other special problems as the need arises. The MS Society has printed a special booklet for families, and it is a good idea for parents and children to read this and to discuss the pictures and comments with each other.

Children's Reactions

While some parents over-protect their children from MS, in other cases the children are involved early on as helpers. They may willingly take on this role but it, too, has its dangers. Children· can grow up to feel guilty about their parent and to feel bad about themselves. If they take on too much responsibility too early in their lives, they may miss out on being cared for and feeling fully loved in their own right. Some children become 'little adults', and this may mean that they fail to grow up normally and may then find it difficult to make relationships later on in life because they remain insecure, or controlling and bossy.

On the other hand, some children react against their parents and will do nothing to help at all. Their way of coping is to cut themselves off from the problem and to try to live as separate a life as possible. Both of these two extremes can be avoided if children are not expected to do grown-up jobs, or to become 'little adults' before they are emotionally ready for this role. Parents need to be aware of these dangers and, while allowing children to help on occasions, it is not right to rely on a child to compensate for the effects of MS, or to let him take on more responsibility than his emotional age and maturity warrant.

I have met several adults who were brought up in a family where one parent had MS. Some of these people have unhappy childhood memories, and of course this is inevitable to some extent. Other 'grown-up' children have found it impossible to help their own parents and feel guilty about what happened. Some have managed to resolve these conflicts by helping other disabled people or by becoming involved with a local branch of the MS Society, where their experience and understanding are invaluable. It is often easier for them to help someone with whom they are less emotionally involved than their own parents, because at times the pain can be too great for them to bear.

Practising for Life
Our two daughters, Clare and Sarah, have settled well in their new home. We have had our ups and downs, but we try to be open and honest with them whilst maintaining our role as the parents who are in charge. This has been difficult at times, but both girls have come to understand my MS by questions and discussion throughout the time that they have been with us. These talks have taken place spontaneously, and over the years they have built up a picture of MS and its implications which they can understand. The girls can now talk openly about MS, and they have met several other people who have the disease, but with different degrees of disability. The picture of a man with MS was drawn by Clare when she was much younger. It is based on her interpretation of my situation and I think that it speaks for itself!

It is necessary for every family to deal with stress of one sort or another, and the more practice that children have in coping with small problems the better they will manage later in life when they have to deal with big ones. Penny and I

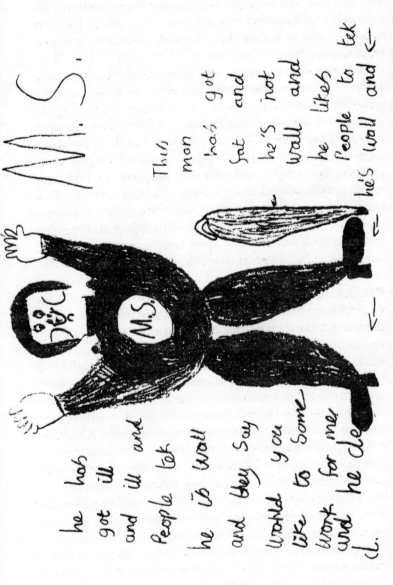

Fig 5. A small child's way of expressing her attitude to MS – a drawing of me by my daughter Clare.

would not have considered taking on Clare and Sarah if my own MS had been worse and if I had not expected to remain reasonably able-bodied for several more years. We are pleased at the way things have worked out and I can see no reason why other families with an MS member should not be able to provide a happy environment for children once disabilities and limitations are accepted as a natural part of life.

I know a woman called Carol whose husband was very severely disabled with MS and who has since died. Carol is a good example of someone who, despite her problems, continued to care for and guide her daughter. Even though her husband was totally paralysed, Carol always tried to share with him decisions about their daughter and always made sure that he, as her father, was fully involved. This must have been difficult to do at times and I admire her greatly. Carol is a genuine expert at living with MS and people like her can teach the professionals a great deal.

In this chapter I may have appeared to dwell too much on the problems that can occur. I have done this because it is important to be aware of these difficulties so that they can be dealt with if they arise and before they get out of hand. But I would like to emphasise that children are often less fragile and more adaptable that they appear. Given plenty of love, understanding and a sense of security, so that they know exactly where they stand, children will not just survive, but grow up to be sensitive and caring towards others. This is not despite their experiences but because of them, and the way that they are handled. Children need to be taught through example; although we cannot choose what happens to us in life, we can choose how we respond to situations. Through them we can learn much about ourselves and about other people, which will enable us to live life to the full, despite the unhappiness and frustration we must all face one way or another along our particular path through life.

9 Professional Help

Although at the moment MS is an incurable disease, there are many ways of helping people and their families to make the best use of their lives, and to adapt to their individual limitations and circumstances. I have already discussed the methods that doctors use to alleviate symptoms. These include steroids for the relief of acute symptoms, and other drugs for the relief of spasticity and to relieve pain. I have also mentioned the importance of a sensible diet and lifestyle.

In addition to these medical treatments, there is a variety of other therapies or services that can help people with their MS, and also their families.

Nursing Care
When MS is diagnosed and the family needs advice, support and further help, most people turn initially to their family doctor. He or she will not only be responsible for the medical management of MS but will also be able to call on other professionals for help, depending upon the needs of the patient. Earlier I examined the doctor/patient relationship and the need for honesty and counselling at the time of diagnosis by both family doctors and neurologists. It is essential that patients are able to trust and to question their doctors throughout the course of the disease, and to receive informed advice, skilled medical care and sympathetic counselling.

Other professionals who may become involved when appropriate include Health Visitors who can offer practical advice as well as counselling, and Community Nurses who can provide support when someone is immobilised by a physical disability. Sometimes they visit daily, to ensure that the patient receives essential nursing care such as the prevention of pressure sores, managing catheters and regulating the bowels.

Nurses play a crucial role, whether in hospital or at home, in making sure that people who are unable to move or to feel pain are regularly moved around and properly cared for. There is no alternative to this regular 'turning', together with trained nursing care, when someone is seriously disabled. In the past people with pressure sores have been taken out of bed and placed in chairs because it was thought that this would allow them to heal. This is not true, for someone who cannot feel sensation or pain can develop serious pressure sores in a chair if he or she is allowed to sit without changing position.

Nurses do a great deal to educate family members about such matters; frequently, they will also be the best people to listen to the worries, fears and frustrations of those who have MS, as well as their relatives. For this reason, nurses need to be trained to listen and to counsel, and they must realise that, although practical help is essential, patients or relatives need to be allowed to ventilate their sad and angry feelings. Inevitably, a good nurse will need to play the part of a counsellor, and she should therefore be trained in counselling skills so that she does not take the anger personally and is able to defuse family tensions in an understanding and constructive way. This is never easy, and I know from talking to nurses how hard they find this part of their work.

Nurses involved in the care and treatment of the severely disabled also need the opportunity themselves to ventilate their own feelings of frustration and anxiety, and for this reason I believe that they, like other professionals, should meet together in regular support groups. These groups should meet frequently and ought not to be seen as a peripheral activity but rather as an essential part of the working week. In this way nurses will feel able to work through their own emotional tensions, and they will be able to care for themselves better. This will also enable them to offer a better service to their patients as well as to their colleagues.

Counselling -What is it?

In the old days, when someone was asked to 'give counsel', advice was expected. The modern word 'counselling' means something completely different and this can be the cause of much misunderstanding. Perhaps the best way of explaining counselling is to examine the different sorts of help that are *not* counselling. I shall do this by listing four possible responses to someone who comes for help with a problem:

1   'You should . . .' This is giving advice, which is not the response of someone who is offering counselling.
2   'If I were you . . .' This is offering an opinion; it is not counselling.
3   'I know how you feel . . .' This is sympathy, not counselling.
4   'I'll sort it out for you . . .' This is offering practical help, which again is not the role of a counsellor.

These four responses will always be useful ways of helping someone, and each will be appropriate on certain occasions, but they are not counselling, because the decisions are being taken by the helping person and not by the person who is being helped. Such responses can make someone feel more helpless and less confident than before, because the helper is in a superior, 'in control', position, while the other person is inferior, 'being helped'.

The essence of a genuine counselling relationship lies in its respect for and attention to the person who has the problem; counselling is a way of allowing a person to help himself. The first skill that a counsellor learns is to listen, the second is to make it clear to the 'client' that he has been heard accurately. After this the relationship is aimed at allowing the client to explore his problems and to clarify his feelings and attitudes to those problems. The counsellor tries to help the client to understand each problem better so that he is able to make a choice or to take action in order to change an unsatisfactory situation. The emphasis should be on the client having responsibility for his own life, by making his own decisions.

Many people are natural counsellors and it is a myth to believe that counselling skills are the exclusive property of any particular professional group. We all use these skills from time to time in our natural relationships with friends or with colleagues at work. In a professional relationship counselling is one-sided because it is part of the service that professionals offer, whether they are nurses, social workers, remedial therapists, psychologists or doctors. Many other professionals use counselling skills and anyone can be trained to improve those that they already have. There are also people who are professional 'counsellors' but they are usually employed to work in a specialist area where they need detailed knowledge as well as an ability to counsel. Counsellors of this sort are sometimes employed by groups of family doctors or in a variety of institutional settings. Some counsellors advertise their services privately, but it would be wise to choose a counsellor carefully under those circumstances because standards vary considerably.

I am not particularly happy about professional counsellors, but I am very keen that *all* professionals who work with people should acquire counselling skills. I see these skills as being just as important as specialist knowledge. For this reason I prefer to encourage health and social care professionals to counsel their own clients rather than taking on the job myself, or suggesting another counsellor elsewhere. Fortunately there is a growing trend for professional people to be interested in counselling and to acquire the necessary skills. I hope that this new trend will one day become the general rule.

Social Workers

Disability often leads to a variety of practical and financial problems, and Social Workers can be invaluable in helping to sort them out. Social Workers can advise on financial benefits, pensions and allowances, they can arrange day and other care facilities, and some may also offer skilled family counselling. The criteria for receiving financial help and other benefits are often complicated and the social worker can explain what a particular person is entitled to, and how to make an application. Details of benefits vary from time to time and it is useful to know where to go to obtain up-to-date information and advice.

In Britain, details of Invalidity Pensions and Disability Living Allowances are available from the Citizens' Advice Bureaux or from the MS Society, as well as from the local Social Service or Department of Health and Social Security offices. Information on these subjects is freely available and I do not intend to go into any one of them in detail. However, I must stress the importance of financial self-sufficiency to any disabled person; this is crucial if he or she is to feel secure and to have self-respect. Many social and relationship difficulties can be alleviated by making sure that families have an adequate income. There should be an appropriate compensation for loss of earned income by a person who has MS, and often another member of the family has to give up her job in order to look after her disabled relative. Financial support will lessen the chances of children having to be received 'into care' and will also allow the family to maintain a reasonable standard of living.

Attitudes to Receiving Financial Help

Assistance of this sort from the State or from the Local Authority is sometimes regarded with suspicion and may be proudly rejected: 'I don't need charity.' This is an understandable response; few of us want to feel that we are dependent on others if we can help it. On the other hand, people should realise that it is not an insult that they are receiving, but in most cases the fruits of their own labour and industry when they were well. There will always be some people who 'work the system for what it is worth', but many go too far the other way and fail to take up assistance to which they are entitled. In the end this is not helpful to other people who are disabled and who cannot afford to turn down the financial assistance that is due to them. Far better for everyone who is entitled to benefits to accept them, because in this way the unnecessary stigma is shared equally and is minimised. Social Security is only a National Insurance System, after all.

I myself have been guilty in this respect, because for a long time I was too embarrassed and proud to apply for a Disabled Person's Orange Badge to help me park my car in privileged positions. It was a social worker friend who eventually gave me full details of the scheme, and who insisted that I apply not only for my own sake, but for the sake of others in a similar situation. He made it clear that the more people let their needs be known, the better it is for everyone with a disability. I waited for a further year after receiving his advice before I eventually applied for the badge. I had changed jobs and was walking less well and I knew that it would be increasingly difficult for me to work or to go shopping without it. The badge has made a great difference to my life, as it has reduced stress and fatigue. This splendid scheme enables many disabled people to live much more fulfilled lives than before.

I went through the same quandary about whether or not to apply for the Mobility Allowance (now known as the Mobility Component of the Disability Living Allowance). I felt that other people deserved it more than I did, and that my income was high enough when compared to that of many others. I also feared that I might be turned down; I have some days when I can walk reasonably well with my stick. On the other hand, there are days when walking is extremely difficult or impossible, especially when the weather is very hot or when I am severely fatigued. In the end I did apply for the allowance and was totally honest about how well I could walk on good days and how difficult it was for me on bad ones. The doctor who examined me was well informed and was aware that MS fluctuates from day to day, and sometimes from one time of day to another. Unfortunately I have heard from many people that some doctors are not so aware of this, and I know people who have been refused the Mobility Allowance unjustly. Most of these have been able to appeal successfully, with the help and support of an MS Society Branch Welfare Officer, a lawyer, the Citizens' Advice Bureau or a Welfare Rights Worker.

Another argument that persuaded me to apply for the allowance was the same one that influenced me in going ahead and requesting the Orange Badge. It was pointed out to me by another person with MS that I had a duty to apply for the allowance, because the more people with MS who did apply and the more the special problems of MS were known, the better it would be for all of us with this particular disease.

The Mobility Allowance has enabled me to travel much more widely and without so much discomfort, fatigue and stress. I am now able to use taxis on occasions where previously I would have attempted to use public transport, despite the difficulties. I have also used the allowance to help me buy a low-geared pedal tricycle; this is a good way of getting down to the shops about a mile from where I live. I cannot walk that far and the tricycle enables me to get around locally without using a car.

Receiving the allowance and having the Orange Badge for parking have made me feel less proud but more human! MS is a great leveller and we who have special needs must stick together and support each other. Instead, I now feel proud that I belong to a country with a sense of social responsibility, and I am glad that people who are handicapped through no fault of their own can receive such assistance and so reclaim their independence and contribute to society. It has been said that you can judge a truly civilised society by the way that it treats its sick and disabled members. This can be summed up in the words 'to each according to their needs, from each according to their ability'. These words are interpreted differently by different cultures, but can anyone deny their good sense or their humanity?

Rehabilitation

This is a word that can have many meanings. I remember shuddering with disgust when I heard that there used to be a Gipsy Rehabilitation Centre near my home. The very idea of 'rehabilitating' gipsies is alien to me. It seems to imply that gipsies are 'abnormal' and 'deviant' and that they must be made to fit in with the rest of society. I admire many of the values and principles that mark the gipsy way of life and I abhor any 'rehabilitation' or 'treatment' that seeks to change other people simply because they are different.

But what about MS rehabilitation? This used to be a one-sided affair, as with the gipsies, but in recent years there has been more emphasis on involving the person who has MS and his relatives in the decision-making central to the rehabilitation programme itself. At a recent seminar on MS Rehabilitation in Switzerland, Margaretha, a Swedish woman who has MS, said the following:

'Rehabilitation includes *any measure* that makes it possible for us to live as normal a life as possible.'

Another speaker, a doctor from Belgium, made it clear that he considered the handicapped person 'not as an ill and separate object of medical attention but as a human being with the potential for growth and development'. A Swiss neurologist defined rehabilitation, as understood by his team, in the following way: 'By the concept of rehabilitation we mean the co-ordinated use of medical, psychological and social measures that help patients to improve as far as possible their physical, mental and social function. Rehabilitation is a learning process not limited in time, which aims at achieving the best quality of life for people with MS.'

The rehabilitation of MS people should also involve their families, friends, work colleagues and, ultimately, the whole community. Instead of trying to change people so that they fit in with the majority, rehabilitation should be seen as team work, with the MS family being the centre of the team. In this way the family is able to take the initiative, to make decisions and to have a large say in the rehabilitation process.

Unfortunately, not all rehabilitation teams function in such an ideal way, but there is certainly an increasing willingness in many parts of the world to try these ideas. This is especially true when people with MS are able to make their own views known at a political level, as is happening now in Sweden.

The Team

Rehabilitation teams vary from place to place, but they will usually include a rehabilitation doctor, occupational therapists, physiotherapists, social workers, psychologists and speech therapists. The rehabilitation doctor co-ordinates the function of the rehabilitation team and the department itself is usually associated with a large hospital, and occasionally with a university. The doctor in charge liaises with family doctors and neurologists, as well as being involved with other members of the team in setting the goals of rehabilitation for a particular patient. The social worker helps to link the family to the department, and will also offer counselling and specialist advice.

The speech therapist can help a person with MS who has difficulty with speaking, as sometimes happens. The aim is to enable the person to adapt to his or her disability, to learn a better technique of pronouncing words and to breathe correctly. Psychologists may be involved in assessing a person's intellectual ability and in setting up behavioural programmes. Sometimes psychologists also offer counselling and conduct group psychotherapy sessions. Some rehabilitation teams may have a counsellor on the staff, but this is not common. In Britain very few consultants in rehabilitation have training in neurology – a pity.

Day Centres

Some rehabilitation centres and teams are sponsored by the MS Society. I quote from a letter that I received from a nurse based at an MS centre in Perth in Western Australia; she describes an interesting and progressive approach to rehabilitation:

The full para-medical team, consisting of two nurses (one at the Day Centre and one doing Home Visiting), a physiotherapist, an occupational therapist and a social worker, has been functioning for twelve months now. There are approximately 350 people with MS in Western Australia and about 80 attend the Day Centre once or twice a week for physiotherapy, occupational therapy, craft activities and socialisation. We also offer yoga, massage, hairdressing and beautician services, the latter two being great morale boosters! A doctor from the Public Health Department, Community Health Section, attends the weekly team meetings in a purely advisory capacity.

The patients in the country areas receive support from their family doctor and the Community Health Centres that have been established in the major regional centres. We hope, by the end of the year, to commence regular country visits by the Home Visiting Nurse to bring the special care and support to these people who cannot have the regular contact with us that their city cousins receive.

We would like to have a psychiatrist or a psychologist to attend the Centre on a sessional basis, to see patients and their families and advise and support the staff.

Day centres in Britain may be provided by a Health Service Rehabilitation Team or by the Social Services. Sometimes a local branch of the MS Society will provide day-care facilities, but this is usually in association with the local Social Services team. Some Young Disabled Units may have day-care provision, as well as hospital beds for those people who are being assessed or who are receiving treatment for the complications of MS.

Who are the people who benefit most from attendance at a day centre? This varies from individual to individual: sometimes a person will require a spell of intensive remedial therapy; someone else might attend for mainly social reasons.

People who live by themselves will benefit from the company of others; those who live with a family can give their caring relatives time to go to work, to go shopping or just to have a well-earned break. Usually there is a mixture of reasons for recommending day-care.

This reminds me of a recent phone call from the wife of someone who has MS. Sylvia told me that she was desperately anxious because her husband, Fred, had become depressed and uninterested in life. He spent all his time eating or watching television at home. He was not practising his physiotherapy exercises and he seemed to have given up all hope. Before the onset of his MS, two years previously, Fred had been running his own business and had spent much time travelling and making important decisions. However, he had eventually been forced to give up his work due to increasing difficulty in walking, and because of fatigue. After stopping work he had quickly lost his own self-respect and also his motivation to get better.

Sylvia had a part-time job and was unable to be at home throughout the day. She felt that Fred had become antagonistic towards her so that, whatever she suggested, he would do the opposite. The purpose of her phone call was to see whether I could 'talk to Fred and make him see sense'. Sylvia seemed truly desperate and said that she was 'at the end of her tether'. It was evident that she had mixed feelings towards her husband: on one hand she realised that she was healthy and that her husband needed to depend on her to some extent, but on the other hand she felt exasperated with him and guilty about her feelings of anger and rejection.

I could understand why Fred might behave in this awkward way. He knew he was dependent on his wife, and yet at the same time he needed to express his anger and resentment at the situation. Deep down he may have felt himself a burden on his wife and wondered whether she needed him any longer. They deserved a break from one another, and Fred needed a chance to mix with others in order to build up his confidence again and to develop new skills. I suggested that Fred might benefit from the local day centre where he would have a change from being at home on his own, and where he could take part in social activities. In this way he might also respond to occupational therapy and his physiotherapy programme could be monitored more effectively. Sylvia would gain from knowing that Fred was not alone and that he was receiving active help and encouragement. It might not be long before Fred developed more independence and regained his self-respect and enthusiasm for life.

It may have helped Sylvia to let off steam on the telephone, but I hope in addition that Fred is now attending the day centre; I am sure that in the end this would help both him and his wife.

10 Occupational Therapy, Physiotherapy and Yoga

OCCUPATIONAL THERAPY

The occupational therapist (OT) is a key member of any rehabilitation team. She may also be based in a hospital department or in the community. Many people with MS never require the services of a full rehabilitation team, either because their disability is only mild, or because they can manage to adapt with help from within their own community. Many of them, however, are helped to come to terms with their disability and to live more fully because of assistance from a community-based occupational therapist.

At a meeting of our MS CRACK self-help group in Andover, one of those present, Mary, who either walks with two sticks or has to use a wheelchair, told us how much help she had received from our local OT, Carolyn. We decided that we would gain a great deal from knowing more about Carolyn's work, and the result was an interesting evening when she spoke to many members of the Andover Branch of the MS Society, together with their relatives, friends and volunteer workers.

She made it clear that occupational therapy aims to help a disabled person to 'achieve his or her own set goals'. These might be mental or physical, or a mixture of the two. She went on to describe how OT began and exactly what her work involved. Many people tease OTs by referring to the making of baskets, and indeed OT did begin as a way of occupying hospital patients by giving them something to do. It helped to take their minds off their situation. But the teaching of basket making, although still important on some occasions, is no longer the main work of a modern OT. They have a three-year training covering many aspects of medicine, surgery and psychiatry and including a year of supervised clinical practice. In Britain, the Chronically Sick and Disabled Persons Act 1970 required local authorities to look to the needs of disabled people in their area and this has led to a number of OTs being employed, like Carolyn, by local Social Services Departments.

Occupational therapy aims to make life easier both for the disabled person and for the caring relative. Sometimes all that is necessary is advice on how to improve everyday techniques, for instance a different way to get into the bath or tips to make shopping easier. Sometimes an OT can provide, free of charge, simple aids such as a raised toilet seat, grab rails near the bath, or hoists. Many aids of this type are also sold by specialist firms and can be viewed in catalogues or at aid centres and bought privately.

The OT can also arrange for the environment to be adapted. It might be necessary for a stair lift to be fitted inside a house or for a ramp for wheelchair access to be built outside it. Occasionally the OT can arrange for an extension to be built on a home or, in the case of council accommodation, for the family to be rehoused in more suitable premises.

The community OT can liaise directly with the Local Authority, as well as with social workers, family doctors and all the other people concerned with rehabilitation. When private houses need to be adapted, grants are sometimes available, but the details vary from time to time and from place to place. People with MS can sometimes benefit from electronic communication aids, especially if their disability is severe. In these cases the OT can contact specialist assessors and help to organise the necessary equipment. Sometimes it is possible to obtain financial help with the installation of a conventional telephone or cordless telephone. If disability is very severe and a person lives in the community, special alarm systems may be provided. These enable the neighbours, the police or the community nursing service to be alerted by the disabled person if an emergency occurs. The local Social

Services Department can also arrange for home helps to visit when a disabled person is living at home, and in some areas a Meals-on-Wheels service is also available.

Wheelchairs

The Department of Health and Social Security (DHSS) through Artificial Limb and Appliance Centres (ALACS) provides a wide variety of wheelchairs. These can be controlled either by the disabled person or by an attendant. Powered wheelchairs are also available for use inside the house and garden, but these are only given to people by the DHSS in special circumstances. At present, only attendant-controlled electric wheelchairs are available in Britain for outside use. Self-controlled electric wheelchairs for outdoor use are available privately, of course, and these are advertised regularly in magazines for disabled people.

Wheelchairs have to be prescribed by a doctor and many factors will influence which is chosen. OTs are trained to assess people's wheelchair needs, and the choice of which chair is suitable for which disabled person is often best left to them. Family doctors who feel that one of their patients needs a wheelchair can refer directly to the OT in the local Social Services Department. OTs take into consideration the environment in which the chair will be used; whether it needs to go into the boot of a car, whether it will go through the door at home, or whether the home will need adapting to suit the wheelchair. Some wheelchairs can be combined with commodes and special light-weight chairs are also available.

Helping the Caring Relative

In her talk about OT, Carolyn emphasised that she tries to help the relatives as much as the disabled person. Relatives who look after a severely disabled person can become exhausted, and are in danger of developing back strain or other injuries if they are not careful. The Crossroads Care Attendant Scheme Trust is a charity that seeks to find and provide care attendants. Many schemes exist and they are often managed by a local charity, such as the Cheshire Homes Foundation, by the Health Authority or by the Social Services Department.

All of these aim to relieve the stress on the caring relative and family by employing a trained person to take over from time to time, and to give the carer a break. This service is now widespread; it can do much to avoid the admission to hospital of a disabled person should the main carer become ill or unable to help for whatever reason. Care attendants do not attempt to replace the statutory Health or Social Services; they are an additional resource.

It is easy to understand the physical and emotional hurt experienced by the person who has MS, but the caring relative is often taken for granted by family members, as well as by Health or Social Services professionals. Both of these groups have a vested interest in the essential caring or nursing that is taking place, and they can sometimes conveniently forget, and fail to take account of, the caring relative's physical and emotional condition.

People often wish to talk to me privately about their personal problems after I have given one of my talks on the psychological and relationship problems of MS. Often it is the caring relatives who need to unburden themselves the most, even more than the people who have MS. I was particularly moved by the following story told me by the wife of a man who was severely disabled by MS. She had been involved in much of the caring required for her husband and had found this exhausting, and often depressing as well. One day at Christmas-time, her husband, in a more than usually depressed frame of mind, had told her that he wished to die, and had asked her if she would arrange things for him. This had been the last straw for his wife; she told me that within twenty-four hours she had been admitted to the Intensive Care Unit of her local hospital suffering from an overwhelming chest infection from which she nearly died. She believed that her sudden illness was due to the emotional turmoil that she had felt when asked to end her husband's life.

I do not know whether this was directly the cause, but I suspect that the emotional conflict which she had experienced, in addition to her already exhausted state, probably played a part in making her vulnerable to an infection and to the serious illness that resulted. This may seem an extreme example, but it does represent the tip of a huge iceberg; we take the caring relative for granted at considerable peril.

PHYSIOTHERAPY

People often hold strong views about the value of physiotherapy in MS: this applies both to those who have the disease and to physiotherapists themselves. Some people with MS are convinced that physiotherapy is the answer to many of their problems, while others think that it does no good at all! This same divergency of opinion exists within the ranks of the physiotherapists, although not quite to such an extreme degree.

I have met physiotherapists who feel that they have much to offer people with MS, but I have also spoken to others who doubt whether they can really help those who have this disease. Some have confided to me that they would be better employed working with the victims of road traffic accidents or with people who have had strokes, because they respond to therapy so much more dramatically.

The truth about the value of physiotherapy in MS probably lies somewhere between these two extremes; although the results may not be dramatic or in any way curative, physiotherapy does seem to have a part to play in the management of MS.

Physiotherapists usually work from a hospital and form part of the wider rehabilitation team I have already described. Therapy can take place in a hospital ward, in the Out-Patient Department, or in a separate clinic. There is also an increasing trend to provide 'Domiciliary Physiotherapy', now more often called 'Community Physiotherapy'. This means that the physiotherapist visits his or her patient at home, rather than expecting the patient to make the journey to the Physiotherapy Department. In this way the physiotherapist can teach and supervise a home exercise programme specially designed for the individual at home and involve family members as well as the patient. Through demonstrating to the relatives what is needed, the physiotherapist can use them as a valuable ally and resource between visits. Often relatives can take an active part in assisting and encouraging the patient with his exercises and so make therapy more effective. Relatives can also be taught the best way to turn the more severely disabled person, and then practice under supervision. People with MS get extra benefit from Community Physiotherapy, because the fatigue and other difficulties involved in travelling are completely abolished. Getting to the Physiotherapy Department can be so exhausting that therapy either becomes impossible due to fatigue, or is so difficult that it is not worth the effort.

Unfortunately, Community Physiotherapy is only available in some areas of Britain, so that many people with MS are completely deprived of this important service. I have been involved in a joint Working Party involving both the MS Society and the Chartered Society of Physiotherapists, which has been set up to explore this unhelpful state of affairs and to judge whether Community Physiotherapy should be made universally available. An additional powerful argument in its favour is the financial one. It is not only more effective as therapy, but is also cheaper in the long term than arranging and paying for complicated transport for people with MS, to get them to and from the Physiotherapy Department.

Benefits of Physiotherapy
What can physiotherapy offer to those of us who have MS? Not everyone will need physiotherapy, especially the many people in whom the disease runs a benign course, but many others can be helped in a variety of ways. Spasticity (stiff legs and arms), for instance, can be reduced through the regular use of certain exercises and by advice on posture when lying

down or sitting up. One technique which is of particular use in MS is based on the beneficial effects of cold. Cold packs or ice towels can be applied to the affected muscles and may reduce spasticity and help to relieve the pain associated with muscle contractures. I know a physiotherapist who reccommends that people who have these problems should keep a large packet of frozen peas for use when required. The peas mould to the area of the body upon which they are placed, and can be frozen again after use ready for the next occasion! (The bag of peas must be wrapped in a damp towel to prevent ice burns.)

I have not tried this method myself yet, as spasticity has not been a problem for me, but I have found that cool baths or a swim in an unheated pool reduce my fatigue and generally improve my mobility and even my vision. Spasticity can also be helped in this way; the benefits are not only due to the cooling of the muscles, but to the general effect of lowering the body's temperature and so improving conduction along the demyelinated nerves (as discussed in the chapter on fatigue earlier in this book).

Of course, it is possible to have 'too much of a good thing' and excessive cold can be harmful and must be avoided. A well-meaning friend of mine with MS recommended cold baths to another friend. The result was disastrous: the person who tried this 'therapy' was made much worse for a while. My own technique is to start off with a luke-warm (but not hot) bath and to run cold water into it until I find it unpleasant but just bearable. I try to stay in the bath for ten minutes and then, re-invigorated, I get out. It is tempting to undo all the good work by warming myself by the fire!

Some Physiotherapy Departments have a hydrotherapy pool which is filled with quite warm water. While it is useful for people with other illnesses, this sort of therapy is best avoided by people who have MS since it may make things worse and bring on fatigue. However, there are always some exceptions, and each individual must find out what temperature suits him or her best. It is possible to experiment with bath water so long as there is somebody ready at hand to help if required.

I myself completely avoid hot baths – and I am not too keen on cold ones, either. The solution for me is to take a luke-warm shower, and I have already mentioned my use of a grab-handle and a strong pole running down the side of the shower, so that I can stand up without falling over, especially when my eyes are shut. In the summer I enjoy the occasional cool and sometimes even cold shower, and I find that this can relieve my fatigue and many of my other MS symptoms for quite a while. Some people find it helpful to keep a stool available to sit on while taking their shower. (A Social Services-based OT may be able to provide this.)

Physiotherapy exercises can be used to strengthen muscles that have fallen into disuse during an MS relapse, and individually tailored exercise and balance programmes can be especially helpful when someone is recovering from a relapse. If a muscle group no longer receives messages due to demyelination in the brain or spinal cord, it cannot respond to strengthening exercises. Instead, therapy will be aimed at strengthening other muscles that the patient may be able to use as an alternative to the disabled ones. When a person has difficulties resulting from tremor and inco-ordination, a physiotherapist can prescribe special exercises involving the use of weights. These can be attached to the wrist, the ankles, and in some cases to the hips. Practising the movements affected by tremor while using the weights can result in a reduction of tremor and an improvement in co-ordination. It is important, however, that these exercises form part of a supervised physiotherapy programme.

Like occupational therapists, physiotherapists are also trained to assess individual requirements for mobility aids and will advise on sticks (canes), walking frames, and wheel-chairs.

Research into helping people with their mobility problems is just as important as finding purely medical ways of treating MS. An interesting new idea being investigated at the moment is whether wearing 'Rocker Shoes' can help certain people who have MS. These are derived from Danish clogs, and there is some evidence that they might help a proportion of people with MS who can benefit from the extra 'push-up' gained from the shape of these shoes, finding that they can walk more normally and with less strain and fatigue. I have seen these shoes and discussed them with people who have tried them. In selected cases they may be effective, but this will become clearer when the research is complete and the results are available for study.

People who have MS respond best to exercise programmes involving short periods of exertion followed by periods of relaxation. The relaxation is just as important as the exercise, and this pattern can also be used successfully in planning the whole day, so adopting a well balanced lifestyle. Physiotherapists are unable to treat patients indefinitely, and anyway this is not necessary, so they usually offer courses of treatment lasting for a few weeks or months at a time. Patients are encouraged, however, to continue the exercise programmes that they have been taught.

THE WHOLE PERSON
The physiotherapist is the ideal person to educate the family on the best use of energy and on the importance of relaxation, and he or she can also prescribe useful exercises to be practised at home, with the help of relatives when necessary. Because they see their patients and their patients' families regularly and often, both physiotherapists and occupational therapists find that they can also listen to the worries and fears that so often beset MS families. Many therapists feel that this part of their work, listening and counselling, is just as important as the therapy itself. They believe that it is necessary to understand the needs of the whole person, and of the whole family, if the therapy is going to have maximum beneficial effect.

There is a danger that some patients and family members will become emotionally dependent on the physiotherapist or

occupational therapist, especially when they provide confident reassurance and authority, characteristic of a caring
parent figure. It is not appropriate for the therapist to take on
the role of a supportive social worker, and an understanding
therapist will have to tread this particular tight-rope
carefully without either rejecting the person concerned, or
letting herself be manipulated and made to feel guilty. This
requires an objective awareness of her relationship with the
patient and the patient's family. Many therapists are
particularly skilled counsellors; a recent survey in Britain
showed that among all health care professionals, physiotherapists were the best at counselling.

Therapists and Doctors

Occupational therapists and physiotherapists often feel angry
with doctors when they are expected to treat someone with
MS who has not been told his true diagnosis. They usually
find that it is much easier to help a person who knows his
diagnosis because it is then possible to explain the reason for
the symptoms and handicaps. The patient is also more willing
to co-operate in therapy. Some therapists have told me that
they are put in an impossible situation when a person asks
them what is wrong, but they are unable to give an honest
reply because the doctor has instructed that the patient
should not know. In these circumstances a therapist may feel
strongly that the person should know the truth, and there is a
risk that the essential two-way communication between her
and the doctor may be jeopardised. Ideally, matters like this
should be discussed at the time of referral so that future
embarrassment can be avoided.

As I stressed in Chapter 4, no one with MS should be kept
unaware of his diagnosis unless there is a very good reason for
keeping him in ignorance. Before any of us can begin to come
to terms with our condition and to do something positive, it is
necessary to know the diagnosis and to understand exactly
what we are 'up against'.

Another frustration that both types of therapist have

discussed with me is that sometimes patients are referred to them too late for maximum benefit. They occasionally feel that both general practitioners and neurologists need to be better informed about the therapies, so that they can think positively and refer earlier. Therapists can feel misunderstood or insufficiently valued and it seems important that they educate doctors about what they can do to help.

Physiotherapy Groups

Some people may prefer to pay privately for physiotherapy, but it is essential first to establish that a physiotherapist offering a private service is properly trained, a member of a professional body, and adequately insured. Some groups of people with MS (whether associated with an MS CRACK group, an MS Society branch, or an MS Therapy Centre) employ their own part-time physiotherapists. This is economically more efficient and the group spirit can also be a beneficial factor when physiotherapy is carried out in this way. I have discussed this way of working with physiotherapists who are employed privately and also with a hospital-based physiotherapist who has set up a similar group in a rural area. The approach lends itself to group exercises, seminars, discussion and self-help. The physiotherapist can provide a focal point for the group and take a neutral role if family relationship problems or doctor-patient issues are brought up, as is so often the case. The main problem with group physiotherapy is that severely disabled people who might benefit are often unable to travel and get readily fatigued. For this reason, these groups are mainly composed of the younger, more recently diagnosed patients with MS, and it may be that the therapy is acting as a useful focus for people who are mostly helping each other with emotional and social problems.

The Future

Most people with MS would benefit from more opportunities for physiotherapy, and many physiotherapists themselves think that their departments are under-staffed and unable to meet all the needs of MS patients. This is especially true for Community Physiotherapy which seems ideally suited to the needs of the more disabled among us. Until it is generally available, many people with MS who might benefit from treatment are being neglected and are not receiving the help to which they are entitled. I for one will not rest until this matter is satisfactorily resolved.

In the meantime, those who wish to help themselves to physiotherapy would do well to study Gill Robinson's book *Multiple Sclerosis – Simple Exercises: A Do-it-yourself Manual*. This can be purchased either from the MSRC, or from the MS Society, who published the book jointly.

YOGA

Once, at a meeting with physiotherapists in London, I inquired whether yoga was regarded as a form of physiotherapy. Opinions were divided, ranging from the view that yoga and physiotherapy had much in common, to the opposite opinion that they were completely different.

My question was not entirely innocent and I had a special reason for asking it. About eighteen years ago, after my first MS symptom but before the diagnosis was confirmed, I was also diagnosed as having 'osteochondritis'. This common but little known complaint occurs mainly in younger people and causes back pain with some limitation of movement in a few cases. My particular trouble meant that I had to be especially careful about my posture or I would end up with a curved spine. I received no regular treatment for this condition but decided to learn some of the techniques of yoga in order to retain a flexible spine as far as possible. Since that time I have carried out a daily routine of yoga postures and I have also used yoga techniques to improve my breathing and my powers of concentration.

A few years later I underwent a spell of physiotherapy following a relapse of my MS. I had lost some of the power in my legs and a certain amount of co-ordination. I discovered

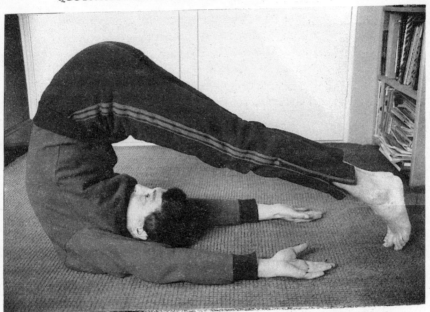

Despite the problems of MS fatigue, it is important to keep fit. I practise my yoga exercises twice a day, and feel much better for them.

that the physiotherapy exercises given to me were very similar to the yoga postures that I already practised! This further encouraged me to pursue my regular yoga sessions.

So *are* yoga and physiotherapy similar, or are they different? The answer must be Yes and No. Yoga is unlike most physiotherapy techniques in that it is derived from an ancient eastern system for promoting physical and mental health. Yoga techniques enable people to have a greater awareness of, and control over the natural powers of their bodies. Yoga is not a religion or a philosophy, and yogis (those who practise yoga) may or may not be religious people. It does not rely upon the supernatural, and the only magic that is involved is the unrecognised magic that lies dormant in each one of us. Neither is yoga a form of sport and it differs from the western concept of exercise because excessive strain is not involved – the emphasis is on balance and rhythm rather than on winning or losing. What is appropriate for one person is not appropriate for another and no competition is involved. For this reason, yoga can be taken up by anyone at any age and at any time, whatever his level of ability or disability.

Yoga offers a 'whole person' approach to health; it sees that the mind and the body are joined together as one. The origin of the word 'yoga' derives from Sanskrit. We have a similar word in our language: 'yoke' – the yoke being what joins two oxen pulling a cart. The aim of yoga is to develop the ability to relax and also to gain greater control over the mind and movements of the body through practising a sequence of rhythmic relaxations and tensions. Correct breathing is one of the first techniques to be learnt by a yogi, and this in itself can release energy and ability that people sometimes never knew existed.

Many branches of the MS Society and MS Therapy Centres organise yoga sessions for their members, and classes should be led by a qualified yoga teacher. In addition, the Yoga for Health Foundation offers weekend and other courses for people who have MS. This charitable foundation is based at Ickwell Bury, a residential centre in Bedfordshire. Yoga is not a cure for MS, but it is a way of increasing potential and discovering hidden resources. Recent research has clearly confirmed that the mind and the body influence each other directly, and that we can do much to manage our MS and to improve our general health through a well balanced lifestyle. Yoga can provide an excellent means to this end and I intend to continue practising both my daily postures and breathing rhythms and my meditation.

Meditation

Meditation can be practised as part of yoga or as a technique in its own right. One group of people in Leeds who have MS combine yoga with an interesting visualisation technique. They first imagine that the demyelination caused by MS in their brains and spinal cords is in the form of blocks of ice. Next they focus rays of warmth on to the ice, and visualise the blocks melting and, at the same time, their illness fading away. Some claim that they feel better as a result. Similar techniques are used by people who have cancer. There is no objective evidence yet that visualisation is effective in suppressing the effects of either illness, but nor is there any evidence that it is useless or harmful. If it reduces tension, gives hope or helps people to feel better, I can see no reason why it should not be encouraged.

You may like to try the following easy to learn meditation technique. It originates in the ancient East and has been the starting point for many seeking to develop their powers of concentration and self-control. The technique can be used as a simple meditation in its own right, or form the basis for further meditation exercises.

First find somewhere comfortable where you can sit upright and where you are unlikely to be disturbed for a little while. You may close your eyes or leave them open as you please. Prepare yourself for the meditation by focusing your mind on your breathing. Be aware of the rhythm of your breathing, how deep or shallow the breaths are, and how evenly or unevenly you breathe in and out. Notice the short periods between breathing in and out, and also between breathing out and breathing in, but do not try to force your breathing in any way. If you are relaxed, your 'stomach' should move out as you breathe *in*, and in as you breathe *out*.

You are now ready to start the meditation. It involves counting each breathing out from one to four, and then starting over again. Count one as you breathe out the first time, and either visualise the number one in your mind, or imagine it spoken aloud in your head. (Whichever you choose, stick to this method throughout the meditation.) Without strain or effort, wait until you breathe out a second time and then count two. Count three on the next expiration, and then four as you breathe out for the fourth time. On the next, fifth expiration count one again and continue counting breaths up to four, before re-starting at number one.

This process sounds very easy but, when you try it, you will probably soon find distracting thoughts or feelings entering your mind. When this happens, be aware of the distractions and let them go. If your counting sequence is interrupted, just start again at one and continue as before. It is very important not to criticise yourself or to feel that you have failed if distractions occur and interfere with the meditation. This very self-criticism is holding on to the distractions and will make matters worse, not better. Besides, there is no right or wrong, no better or worse, but just 'what is'. Meditation is non-competitive and, whatever happens, you just need to be aware of it, and then to go back to the sequence. It is also a distraction to feel smug about how successful you have been. In meditation, pride is a distraction and, in the words of the proverb, it precedes a fall! Continue the breath-counting meditation for five minutes initially, and then stop.

If you want, you can practise this meditation regularly and extend the time by a further five minutes as you get used to it. Sometimes it will be much easier than at others, but after regular practice you may be able to continue for twenty minutes or more. The effects will be beneficial and will lead to better concentration and memory, as well as a general improvement in relaxation and self-confidence. Eventually you will be able to use this technique in all sorts of situations, from waiting on a station platform to travelling in a bus. Some people find that they can regain peace and tranquillity through this technique if they are upset, anxious or angry about something. Others find that it helps them to get their lives in perspective, and some use it as a prelude to sleep.

Many types of meditation are available, but the one that I have described is a good basis for other, more demanding techniques. If you master the breath-counting meditation, you will always have a useful technique and skill when you need it. Some will wish to go further and to explore more powerful techniques, but for most people this is not necessary. So why not try the breath-counting meditation and see how it can help you?

11 Fulfilment and Self-respect

Away from Home

Sometimes people with MS need to be admitted to hospital or to other residential settings which cater exclusively for those who are disabled. Special treatment may be necessary in order to deal with complications of the disease such as pressure sores or urinary infections. On other occasions admission may be required to ensure a full assessment of a person's physical, emotional and social needs, and so that a tailormade rehabilitation programme can be planned. Doctors, nurses, therapists and social workers will be able to observe problems at first hand and can then co-ordinate the best possible solution to the difficulties experienced by a particular individual and his or her family.

Other residential settings can provide opportunities for a person with MS to rest, build up strength and learn new ways of coping with the disease. Short-term care can often enable a strained marriage to survive and families to stay together by giving a break both to the person with MS and to the relatives. Sometimes a short period of residential care is all that is needed, but on other occasions planned 'intermittent' care or even long-term care will be the best policy.

I have not been admitted to hospital in connection with MS, but there was an occasion not so long ago when I was able to discover for myself what it can be like living away from home in accommodation especially adapted to the needs of people with MS. My story begins somewhere in the Highlands of Scotland . . .

I was in a large yellow ambulance with 'The Multiple

Sclerosis Society' written on the outside in bold, black letters. I was accompanied by a nurse – in plain clothes, I might add – and being driven by a policeman, also in plain clothes. We were miles from anywhere surrounded by mountains and I was suddenly struck by the humour of the situation. A psychiatrist, a policeman and a nurse – it sounded like one of those jokes – or perhaps we were in a TV melodrama all set to take part in some sort of exciting life-and-death sequence on behalf of the secret service? No, we were there for more mundane reasons. I had been the guest speaker at the AGM of the Aberdeen branch of the MS Society on the previous night, and I was being taken in the ambulance to Holmhill, an MS Society holiday centre, where I was to give another talk. The plan was for me to stay there for the night before returning home the next day. The nurse was a committee member of the Aberdeen branch, and the policeman was off duty, giving up his time to help the branch as ambulance driver.

I was apprehensive about the holiday centre. It was specially geared to the needs of people with MS and catered for some severely disabled people. I was to stay there as a guest, but because I had MS myself, I was worried in case I should be labelled and treated as 'a patient'.

I had spent the night before at Aberdeen in a special hostel for disabled people, rather than in a hotel. The choice had been mine, but the idea of finding out about this sort of special accommodation at first hand appealed to me. On that occasion I had also been anxious about what I might find; I was concerned about losing my personal identity and being classed as 'one of the disabled'.

As it turned out, I need not have had such fears. The Margaret Blackwood Housing Association was an excellent example of how the special needs of people who are disabled can be met, without making them feel second-class citizens or freaks. Some of the residents had MS and I had an opportunity to talk to them and their partners. I found that most of them were living full and 'normal' lives within the limits of their disability and they were pleased to be in accommodation adapted to their individual requirements. Some lived in houses with gardens, together with their partners and children; others were the proud occupiers of self-contained flats, easy to maintain and fully adapted for their needs. People who were more severely disabled lived in a hostel where they had their own rooms; meals were provided for them and they had assistance when necessary from the friendly and skilled helpers.

I enjoyed my stay there and was pleased to see that the staff were not fussy and over-protective, but that instead they encouraged the residents to be as independent as possible. Many residents were thus enabled to have a larger say in the running of their own lives than might otherwise be possible. They also had privacy and, because of these things, they seemed to have maintained a normal sense of self-respect and respect for others.

So, as we neared the Holmhill Holiday Centre in the Highlands, I began to wonder whether it would be as enlightened as the Margaret Blackwood Centre or whether it would be a 'them and us' situation. Them – staff; us – patients! How disabled would the other people be? Would the atmosphere be 'nursy' and hospital-like, or would relationships within the centre be equal, with respect for the individual rather than an over-emphasis on illness and disability?

Well, once again, it turned out that my fears were groundless. Most of the residents (not called patients) were there for a two-week break and they certainly seemed to be having a good time. The weather was fine and the hot sunshine was almost too much for those of us with MS who do not like to be heated up too much! The staff were understanding and without being too pushy provided a range of options for the residents who were neither patronised in a jolly way or patted on the head and shoved in a corner. The day before my arrival some of the residents had been on a whisky tasting visit to a local distillery, and on the afternoon that I came several were relaxing and chatting quietly while sipping cool drinks.

Holmhill is a very busy place and normally it is not possible for relatives to stay there as well. But there are other holiday opportunities where it is possible for the whole family to go away together, with adequate facilities being provided for the disabled member. This can suit some families better.

Long-term Residential Care

Sometimes people with MS have to accept longer-term residential care or treatment, and this can be a frightening experience. Initially there can be mixed feelings of relief and guilt from their families, coupled with feelings of relief but also of rejection from the one who has MS and has been obliged to leave home. Some people will live for the rest of their lives in residential care, perhaps in one of the Cheshire Homes or in a hospital unit. On one occasion I visited a hospital unit for the young disabled which provided both short-term and intermittent care as well as long-term care for a whole range of people with severe disability or chronic illness. The nurses at this unit were keen to help the residents become more fulfilled and independent. This is not an easy thing to do because it requires money, plenty of time and skilled staff who are supported by positive long-term policy decisions made by the managing authorities.

Although I was impressed by the staff's desire to give the residents more freedom and autonomy I was disappointed to learn that sometimes this practice was being undermined. One of the nurses illustrated the problem with the following story. A young man in her unit regularly enjoyed looking at the Page 3 nude pin-up in his daily newspaper. He had stuck one of his favourite pictures on the wall beside his bed. The nurse felt that this was a normal and healthy thing for him to do and that it might help him to cope better with his unnatural situation. But a doctor came by and ordered the nurse to have the picture removed.

This angered me because I feel that if someone is going to

need long-term care in such a place, at least the surroundings can be made to feel homely and as personal as possible. Residents should have the privacy that they need as well as autonomy over the choice of decoration, furnishings and the lay-out of their room or their area in the ward. It can have done nothing for this young man to be deprived of his pin-up, except to make him feel more powerless and even more of a third-class person than before.

Some feminists might be offended at the idea of men enjoying themselves looking at nude pin-ups, because this can possibly be seen as humiliating to women. But in this case we are concerned with a different issue, the issue of choice for the young man. It is not a question of whether his choice is sexist or even immoral. The doctor's objection might have been that the pin-up would be sexually overstimulating for the young man, or might upset the other residents. But these are matters that the young man himself and the other residents should decide, not the doctor who should be there to serve the needs of his patients and not to 'play God.'

Attitudes to residential care are changing and there is reason to be optimistic about future trends. People who work in this field are more than ever aware of the need to treat their patients or residents as individuals and give them respect and dignity. At one hospital unit I was impressed to find that the residents had almost total privacy. Their rooms were fitted with lockable doors and there was provision for a partner to come and stay the night if they liked. In this way the natural sexual needs of the couple could be met, as well as the simple need for them to be on their own together at times. In this particular unit, staff and residents had to knock on the door before going into a person's room.

It is not always easy to run this enlightened type of residential care. The staff must have regular support groups so that they can meet together to give time to their own needs and deal with the many frustrations and misunderstandings that can occur, both in their relationships with residents and with each other. But because it is difficult and expensive to run such a unit is not a reason for not trying. We must continue to air these matters openly and work for more units of this sort, and to improve the standards of the residential units that are already in existence. In this way people who have to live in residential accommodation can retain and develop a sense of self-respect and control over their own lives.

Living in the Community

Maintaining self-respect when people with MS live away from home is often difficult, but neither is it easy for those who wish to live fulfilled lives in the community at large.

A young man with MS was on holiday with his wife in one of the more remote and rural corners of Europe. She was pushing him in his wheelchair through the narrow streets of a small market town when they met an old woman, draped in a long black shawl, coming the other way. Evidently the woman was dismayed by what she saw, for she seemed to look anxiously about her as if hunting for an escape route. Not finding one, she had to pass close to the fearful object in her path. My friend, the man with MS, told me afterwards that he was amazed to see her make a religious sign as if to protect herself from the evil eye and then, as she went by, she slipped him a few coins before hurrying away!

This experience left a lasting impression on the man and his wife. They knew that they had witnessed something very primitive, but that nonetheless it represented something all too common in society, although usually manifested in a more sophisticated way. They saw in what had happened a symbol of what frequently occurs when someone who is disabled meets a 'normal' or able-bodied person.

The old woman had probably been taken unawares and, faced with a young disabled man in a wheelchair, she had reacted to her anxiety and fear in a ritual fashion which made her feel better. The religious sign was a way of magically protecting herself against the apparition in case she should be contaminated by the evil forces she imagined might be present! The giving of money was her way of making a sacrifice to the gods; rather like paying an insurance premium against becoming disabled herself. It could also be seen as a way of coping with the guilt of being able-bodied when in the presence of someone stricken by fate. She was not only keeping on the right side of the powerful and unpredictable gods but was also paying off a debt; she could then safely pass by and forget my friend with MS – she had 'done her bit'.

The old woman's response was probably well-meaning, but it was based on the fear and ignorance about disability that lurks within us all to some degree. What she did represents society's response throughout the world to people who are disabled. Guilt money is paid to charities and the ritual flag of protection against the evil eye is placed on the lapel! The ritual completed and the money given, people who are disabled are expected to be grateful and not to complain. They will be looked after. They will be provided for, given holidays, taken out and generally patronised. It is almost as if society is saying, 'Let's keep them separate; let's keep them out of sight; don't upset other people.' Perhaps I have exaggerated, but certainly this is the attitude of many people. Of course, giving money to charities helps those who are unable to work or to provide for themselves, but this should not be an excuse for remaining ignorant or for not 'becoming involved'.

There is a danger that people who have MS will find themselves being buried under a heap of charity money and good works. They can be prevented from making decisions, taking responsibility for themselves, or from making a contribution to others. It sometimes seems that they must not give, because they are there so that other people can use them, in order to make themselves feel good and generous! The effect upon those who have MS can be disastrous. They are made to feel useless, a burden on society and to have no positive role or function.

Another way that people behave when faced with someone who has MS is to pretend that it is not happening. They try not to see, not to accept the suffering or disability that is in front of them, and this denial of reality is also alienating to those of us who are disabled. This denying behaviour seems to imply that we, who have MS, lack 'will power' or 'moral fibre' and that we are as we are because of our own personal weakness, or even wickedness.

I came across an example of this type of behaviour when I was walking down the High Street of my own home town in the south of England, minding my own business. Suddenly there was a shout from the other side of the street, and I saw a man I did not know pointing and waving at me. He shouted again and came across the road to talk further. 'Young man,' he said, 'you don't need that stick – you can walk without it. I will buy it off you for one pound.'

I declined his offer, feeling rather embarrassed, and definitely some sort of a freak. He pressed his point, but in the end I walked away from him having first made it clear that I had a disease called MS which made my legs weak, and that my stick was a great help to me.

This experience made me feel guilty about having a stick, and I must say that, deep down, his offer had attracted me. I had almost believed for a moment that his magic would cure my MS and that if I sold him the stick I would not need it. I had succumbed to the same denial of reality that the man in the street needed in order to cope with me. Afterwards I laughed and got things a little better in perspective. Once again I knew that I had witnessed something that happens all the time to people who have MS. I had been alienated, rejected and used by someone who could not cope with having to accept the real me. This man had tried to reject me and to deny that I was in need and disabled.

On another occasion, when I was on my way to an MS meeting, I came across a group of teenagers at a railway station. They looked embarrassed to see me, and one of them shouted out bravely, 'Hello, Grandad!' He looked for a response from his friends who laughed and walked on.

This is yet another way that society deals with people who are disabled. The boy had coped with his anxiety and fear by making a joke. This seemed to give him strength and to make him feel better, but it was at my expense. My momentary anger gave way to understanding and forgiveness once I realised that he was a young lad growing up and trying to make sense of a strange world. MS is sometimes very frightening to other people.

Recreation

These stories illustrate the need for those of us with MS to take as full and active a part in society as we are able. But it is easy to feel demoralised and to avoid mixing with able-bodied people because it sometimes does not seem worth the effort.

People with MS who are unable to work for whatever reason can often find ways to increase their confidence and sense of fulfilment by taking part in recreational pursuits. Sports for the disabled are more available now than they used to be, and they can help people not only to achieve a sense of satisfaction and a feeling of success, but also to enjoy themselves and simply have good fun! Many of us feel better after exercise, especially if we can pace ourselves and acknowledge our own limits. Fatigue, of course, is always a problem and allowances have to be made for adequate rest periods. Sports can increase self-confidence generally and help people who have tended to be isolated at home to become more fully integrated with the able-bodied community.

I have personally enjoyed horse-riding on occasions but, unfortunately, this recreation has left me shaken up and extremely tired afterwards. I have always needed a good rest in order to recover from riding and these days I seldom do it. More useful to me is a swim in a cool pool. Swimming helps me to feel good because the differences that mark me out from other people physically are less pronounced. It can be especially pleasing when I find that I am actually able to swim faster than my able-bodied friends! I also feel much more lively after a swim, and I can be revived from severe fatigue in this manner, possibly because the cool water has lowered my body temperature and improved the conduction of messages along my nerves. I certainly see and walk better for a while.

I have already mentioned the tricycle which I obtained with my Mobility Allowance. I enjoy riding this because it is safer from the balance point of view than an ordinary bike and because I can sit on it and talk to people over their garden hedges without getting off and having to stand up! My own particular tricycle was custom-built and has specially lowered gears. This enables me to pedal more easily up slopes. I also have a holder for my walking stick and toe caps which stop my feet falling off when I get tired. I do not go long distances on my tricycle, but it *is* exercise, and I enjoy the independence and the feeling that I am giving myself physiotherapy as I go along.

Most of us need hobbies and interests as well as exercise and sport. These also help people who could otherwise be stuck at home to meet others who may or may not be disabled but who share similar interests. It is particularly important for people who are unable to get out and have a change from home. These pursuits can be mentally stimulating and they also help the able-bodied members of society to see people who are sick or disabled as basically like themselves, with similar needs and ways of enjoying life.

It is important that people who have MS are helped to be as independent as possible with respect to mobility and access to buildings, and it is good to see that there is an increasing use of self-powered wheelchairs and motor tricycles. In Britain the Mobility Allowance has undoubtedly helped housebound people to achieve greater independence and self-reliance.

Work

Many people with MS work normally, despite their disabilities; this is encouraging because sport and leisure interests (however helpful they may be) are no substitute for work. Work is the ultimate way of feeling fulfilled and

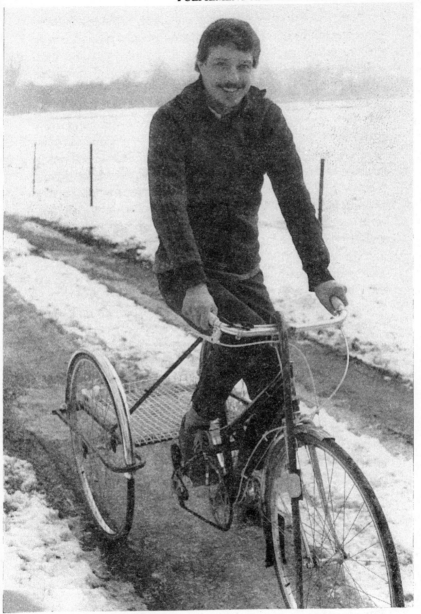

For longer trips, my low-geared tricycle has proved invaluable. It's good exercise, too.

anything less, however satisfying, will rarely provide the same sense of fulfilment and self-respect. People who are not working often feel that they are second-class citizens, and some, sadly, even have a sense of being parasites on society. It is therefore essential to do everything in our power to make it possible for people to work, whatever their limitations. This may well involve adapting the place of work, changing work patterns, or making other allowances for the person with MS. Rest periods may be necessary for those who experience fatigue, and if full-time work is not possible, then part-time is the next best thing. Unfortunately, benefits and sick-leave are not geared to part-time work plans, and society generally seems to have an 'all or none' attitude to work. Either you are one hundred per cent fit and work full-time or you are 'sick' and work not at all. We need to make employers and others in society more aware of this nonsense which divides people up too neatly.

We are all individuals, and we have to strive to make sure that our individual needs are met so that we can contribute in our own individual way. Work enables us to feel a sense of self-satisfaction and achievement. It also gives us independence and helps us to feel that we are recognised as useful citizens, as well as enabling us to be financially self-sufficient. This in turn creates the ideal conditions for further independence and autonomy. A possible vicious circle is broken once somebody is working; the alternative is for a gradually escalating sense of helplessness, dependency and loss of self-esteem. Work means, too, that people can develop new skills, adjust better to their disease and increase their participation in the community. It means that people with MS do not feel so stigmatised or different from the able-bodied and this can only encourage greater integration throughout all the various levels of society.

Overcoming Problems
There are many reasons why a person with MS might have difficulty continuing to work. Problems with vision or co-

ordination can make some types of work impossible, and a hot environment will exacerbate the symptoms of MS fatigue. There may also be difficulties in getting to work, and the work place may not be easily accessible, or it might not be adapted to the special needs of the disabled person. For instance, the lavatory may be upstairs and difficult or impossible to reach. Psychological symptoms such as poor concentration or memory problems may also affect a person's ability to work, and lack of confidence and self-respect can be associated with depression, low morale and fear of change.

Most countries have ways of helping disabled people to continue or to obtain work, and in Britain the Manpower Services Commission (MSC) is active in this area. They provide information for employers on many aspects of disability, ranging from how to obtain help to adapt the work place, to ways of re-training disabled employees. The MSC, in conjunction with the MS Society, has produced a useful leaflet for employers about the employment of people with MS.

In the local community it is the Disablement Resettlement Officer (DRO) who deals with the individual problems of people who are physically handicapped, and who also works with local employers. He or she can carry out an assessment of a person's employment needs and abilities and may call upon the medical or social work professions for help with this. The DRO advises on how best a person with a disability can adjust to work and, in some cases, can provide financial help with fares and transport. The DRO can also arrange for employers to have grants to cover the expense of adapting the work place for an employee who develops MS. In cases where this would not be helpful, he or she can alternatively arrange for a person who has MS to undergo re-training and change to another, more appropriate job. It is also possible to obtain special aids, such as an electronic typewriter, when these are required by a disabled person.

In Britain Nicole Davoude, who founded the MS CRACK groups, has made a special study of the employment of people who have MS. In particular she has pointed out the obstacles to employing someone part-time. She has suggested that the government might establish a 'State of Partial Incapacity' and so enable many people with disabilities to be employed part-time without a loss of financial benefits. Nicole noted that employers often have a negative attitude towards taking on people who are disabled, and that trades unions are also sometimes suspicious. She and others from the MS Society have done much to publicise these points and to lobby Members of Parliament. There is no reason why a diagnosis of MS should also mean a future of unemployment. Being employed part-time myself, I know how important this can be. As a doctor, I am fortunate in being able to work for six half-days a week, and to have sufficient income for my own needs. But for many at the moment, part-time work is financially uneconomic, even if the opportunities existed.

If for any reason it proves impossible to obtain outside work, then it is worth exploring the possibilities of work that can be done at home. Good typists are always in demand, and many offer employment to people who will sell goods or co-ordinate services by telephone. Home computers are another possibility, and quite a number of disabled people have created work for themselves in this field. Publishing houses may need help with proof-reading or reviewing books. Other opportunities are there for people who are prepared to look for them.

Many women may see their proper work as looking after their home and family. They may find that disability interferes with this role and become frustrated at having to rely increasingly on their relatives to help with the shopping and cooking. Most families are willing to help, but it can be annoying not to be able to choose for oneself – especially personal items, such as clothes or make-up.

Several firms offer a wide range of goods by post, and shopping this way is far less tiring. It enables the person with MS to make his or her choice of items at leisure, without the hassle of going to the shops. Home-buying parties of the kind run by 'Tupperware' and 'Orlane' are sometimes criticised, but they do enable some people with MS to get out, to do their shopping in an easy way, and to enjoy a social occasion. Many hairdressers are willing to come to the house of a disabled person. All this can help someone to maintain personal pride in her appearance, which goes hand-in-hand with self-respect.

Even the most disabled woman can still feel an important part of the family if she remains in charge of planning meals and making suggestions for the shopping list. She may be able to teach her husband or children to cook and she can play an active part in planning the day-to-day running of the household. It is important for families to encourage this kind of contribution.

After the first printing of this book, some people wrote to say that I should have mentioned the value of non-MS voluntary work. They emphasised how important it is to be fulfilled in *work* that is useful, interesting and possible even when paid employment is no longer possible. I agree: there are lots of opportunities to do voluntary work locally and it is rewarding and very necessary. Working for Greenpeace, the British Legion, the Samaritans or a political party are some ideas to think about – there is always a cause to support or something to protest about, and some of us need to get away from disability occasionally!

Postscript: Creating Meaning

'Physician, heal thyself!' There is something disturbing about a sick doctor. Perhaps it does not seem quite right that those who say that they can heal others should become ill themselves. The implication behind this view is that doctors who are sick are unlikely to be much good at treating the medical problems of other people. A sick doctor! What can he do for us if he cannot help himself?

It may be for this reason that many doctors try to hide their own illnesses, and sometimes present a false image. Perhaps they fear a loss of credibility if they admit that they, too, are mortal! I have often heard stories about colleagues who have turned up for work with heavy colds, or some other illness, only to find that they are worse than many of their patients! I have been guilty of this myself and, despite coming to terms with my MS symptoms, there are occasions even now when somehow I feel unable to care for myself properly. It is as if some of us doctors need sick people to treat in order to feel useful and important, but when we are stricken with illness ourselves we are unprepared, and sometimes unable to cope. I have certainly learnt my lesson the hard way over the years and am now much more able to admit to being unable to work properly when I feel ill. It has taken me a long time to reach this state, and I still feel uneasy and guilty when I am at home or in bed, because a part of me feels that I should be working and at the service of my patients. I now realise that my ability to accept my own mortality and my own vulnerability is actually helpful to my patients; it is important both for them and me to realise that I am not indispensible, and that if tomorrow I am run over by a bus and killed, the world will continue much as before.

But there is a more positive aspect to the sick doctor: a healer who has personally experienced the grip of the gods and the unfairness of fate can be a healer with increased powers. Contact with the gods, however painful, may offer us an experience that profoundly alters the way that we see things and the way that we live our lives. When a doctor has been seriously ill or is disabled, he or she can never be the same again. The experience of illness, of loss, of uncertainty about the future or of impending death, can free a person from previously held illusions and prejudices, and from a narrow view of life. This may enable a doctor to turn into a healer; or to put it another way, it can be the catalyst that allows the textbook expert to transform himself into a caring and understanding physician.

I believe that having MS myself has helped me to become more sensitive to the needs of others and that it has enhanced my skills as a healer. In my own case, illness came to me at the same time as my medical training and I often think of myself as being doubly qualified, firstly as a patient and secondly as a doctor – the order is important! Through having MS, I have had to face my own frailty and mortality. It has been painful at times and the reality has not been easy to bear. I have known periods of deep depression and a feeling of hopelessness and despair. I have come through these black nights and I have become familiar with many of the devils that inhabit my particular hell.

Meeting the devils and finding a path through the forest of life is a universal experience, for this is a journey that we must all make. For me, MS has been a major devil. This book is a record of my attempts to understand and grapple with MS and to find the best way forward. I no longer ask, 'Why me?' I know that MS is my special challenge and that life is unfair to everyone in different ways. Moreover, I now know that life is not only unfair, but that the events that occur are often in themselves random and meaningless. That is, until we give these events some meaning, for it is only when we can look the gods in the eye and answer 'Yes' to life that we can begin to take responsibility for ourselves, to accept whatever fate brings us and to make the most of it. If we cannot or do not act in this way we may spend our lives seeking answers where they cannot be found, or blaming our suffering and unfair lot either on the gods or on other people. We all have a variety of different challenges to face: these are the questions that are asked of us by life, and we have to answer and respond, whether we are the parents of a mentally handicapped child, a bereaved husband or wife, or dying from cancer in a hospital ward.

I hope that I have used my experience of MS in order to understand myself and to cope better with what often seems an unfair and sad world, yet which is at the same time a mysterious and wonderful one. I think that I am now at last beginning to say, in my more positive moments, 'Why not me?' This gives me a sense of peace and acceptance. I realise that I am part of this universe, part of the natural world. I no longer need to fight because I know that I have the power in me to respond to whatever has to be. Although I cannot change the cards that life has dealt me, I do have some choice about how I play my hand, about how I answer my fate.

Up until now my challenge has not been as difficult as that which faces many people who have MS, and I sometimes wonder whether my philosophy would hold up under less favourable circumstances. Would I still be able to write these words if my MS were worse and if support from family and friends were lacking? If we are to create meaning in our lives then we have to make decisions, take risks and be responsible for choices, however limited these may be, or however enormous their implications. We either cast ourselves adrift at the mercy of the oceans or we make an attempt to respond to our fate by accepting our limits, and then by using the potential we still have. This is living.

We can decide to use what is left of our abilities in order to create some meaning from our experiences, both for ourselves and those around us. For me, this is the only answer to the question of suffering and unfairness that life has placed before me. This is an answer to life, not a question, and it helps me to live with hope and to collaborate with the gods in creating meaning in a world that can otherwise seem hopeless and unfair. Whoever or wherever we are, we are part of nature and we have a role to play, however small our part may sometimes seem. In this way we can live NOW, in the present, as fully as possible, glancing neither backwards nor seeking to look too far into the distance ahead of us.

This book has not given easy answers on how to live with MS and it would be ridiculous to pretend that any such answers exist. I have instead recorded my own journey through that part of the frightening and mysterious territory of MS in which I have found myself. I hope that this record will act as a guide book or map for others who travel along similar paths.

Appendices

1 SOCIETIES ASSOCIATED WITH MS

The Multiple Sclerosis Society

This is the main voluntary organisation which cares for and supports people and their families who have MS. It is also concerned with raising money for research into the disease.

For many years I kept well clear of anything to do with the MS Society. This was partly due to the fact that it took me a long time fully to accept that I had the disease, and partly because I did not want to be associated with people who were more severely disabled than myself. I also thought that the Society consisted of unbearable 'do-gooders' or 'Lady Bountifuls' who either needed to look after other people, or who did voluntary work in order to advance their social status in the community.

I did eventually decide to join the MS Society once I had accepted that I was disabled and that I would have to make adjustments to my life, such as working part-time. I thought that, as a doctor who had been through the early traumas of MS, I would be able to offer something to other people.

One evening I got out the telephone directory and discovered that the nearest branch of the MS Society was in a city twenty miles away from my home; with some degree of apprehension I rang the number. I soon found myself talking to the Welfare Officer of the Southampton Branch. She insisted on coming to see me at my home and, without more ado, a date was fixed. I waited apprehensively for her visit. Then I noticed a large van parking outside and two people emerged. (I afterwards discovered that this van was referred to as 'the transport'.) My next impression was of an elderly couple, both warm and friendly in their manner, standing in my doorway.

They were soon talking to Penny and me in our living room. Both of them were kind and compassionate, but I was rather disconcerted to find that they were quite old, and in different ways they were disabled themselves! Mr Lockyer told me that he had survived a heart attack, and his wife was troubled by arthritis and had some difficulty with walking. Despite their age and their disabilities, they came across as two charming people who were keen to help me. Their sincere wish to be of service frightened me and I had to make it clear that we did not want to be helped, but to help others. After a while Mr and Mrs Lockyer accepted this fact, but they remained determined to provide us with transport so that we could attend the next social meeting.

Initiation
When the day came we were picked up by a tall, middle-aged lady who turned out to be a voluntary nurse from the St John's Ambulance Brigade; she was also a member of the branch committee. We both enjoyed talking to Miss Maltby on the way down to Southampton. She had a good grasp of MS and a wide experience of helping people with the condition, but she was not at all patronising in her manner.

The meeting was in a large hall, especially built for disabled people and containing rows of tables and chairs. There were severely disabled people present; some were in wheelchairs, others had crutches or sticks, but there were not many people like me, with only slight disability. It seemed to be what they wanted – a chance to get out, to play bingo and other games and to have a chat and something to eat and drink. However, Penny and I did not really feel that it was our scene! The committee of the branch cleverly took advantage of this, and of the fact that I was a young doctor prepared to play a part in the Society. I discussed with them the fact that there were very few newly diagnosed and less disabled people present and it was not long before we had started Southampton's first MS CRACK group.

Penny and I had been initiated into the MS Society, and although thrown in at the deep end, we decided that we could play a part in its future. At that time no one with MS was on the local committee and, in common with several other branches of the Society, it was considered inappropriate for people who actually had MS themselves to serve. It was thought that they might hear something distressing, or alternatively, they might be emotionally over-involved, and therefore would not be able to make proper judgements.

This attitude did not please me and I am glad to note that, since I joined the Society, attitudes have changed dramatically. It is now common practice for people with MS to serve on branch and national committees of the MS Society and they take an increasingly active part in the running of the Society. Although I am impressed by the changes, there is still quite a long way to go. I should like to see even more participation by people with MS than there is at present. Sweden and Canada, for instance, have a large proportion of people with MS in their MS organisations and committees.

History
The MS Society in Britain was originally founded by the late Sir Richard Cave at a meeting held in 1953, and from that time it has gone from strength to strength. Sir Richard (who was then plain Mr Cave and who worked at the House of Lords) received a phone call from an unknown American lady. She summoned him to a breakfast meeting with her at 8.30 am the next morning, at the Savoy Hotel in London. He was told that she could give him only three quarters of an hour! He got up early, went to London for the meeting, and met the American lady. Her name was Miss Sylvia Lawry.

She said that she had started an MS Society in the USA and she suggested that he was the man to do the same thing in Britain. She was aware that his wife had MS and she told Mr Cave that her own brother also suffered from the disease. He had MS in a progressive form and he had not experienced any remissions. Miss Lawry knew that other people did have remissions in MS, and she wanted to learn as much as she could to help her brother. In 1945 she had placed an advertisement in a national newspaper requesting information from or about people with MS who had experienced remissions. There was a large response, and it was from these contacts that Miss Lawry founded the National Multiple Sclerosis Society of the USA in 1946.

Mr Cave was impressed by Miss Lawry, and the outcome was a small meeting in the House of Lords, followed by a great deal of work. He went on to found the Multiple Sclerosis Society of Great Britain and Northern Ireland. At the beginning it was not always easy. John Walford, the present General Secretary of the Society, attended one of the more disastrous attempts to publicise the movement in its early stages. A large publicity function, complete with food and drink, was put on in order to introduce the MS Society to the public. Mr Cave, John Walford and many important people were there to meet the media, but not one of the journalists who had been invited bothered to turn up. It was a total flop, but not without its funny side!

This disappointing and difficult start contrasts with the present-day MS Society which is run on professional lines by the small staff at the London headquarters, and with minimal administration costs. The Society now raises and spends millions of pounds each year on research, as well as on the welfare needs of its members.

The International Scene
Miss Lawry is at present the Founder Director of the National MS Society of the USA and Sir Richard was the Founder President of the British MS Society. Due to their efforts and to those of many other people, there is now an International Federation of Multiple Sclerosis Societies (IFMSS). Delegates from all the National MS Societies meet annually to share knowledge about research, welfare, publicity and fund

raising, and to encourage the formation of new MS Societies in other countries.

When I first attended one of these meetings as a delegate of the British MS Society, I was both surprised and disappointed to find that few people who had MS were active in the work of the IFMSS or on its committees. Things have changed since then, and over the last few years several of us with the disease have increased our involvement at international conferences, despite the problems of fatigue and disability that make travelling so difficult. We now play an influential part in the decision-making of the IFMSS at all levels, through our workshops for people with MS, and through the meetings of Persons with MS International (PWMSI). These activities not only 'educate' professionals about the problems of having to live with MS but also encourage the formation of self-help groups and greater participation with national MS societies.

The MS Society in Britain

The backbone of the British MS Society is its system of local branches, and there are now more than three hundred and fifty of these scattered throughout the country, run by volunteers who are supported by the small headquarters staff in London. The branches are the 'front line' of the Society and the people who work in them are in day-to-day contact with the whole range of problems that can occur in MS families. Branches, although autonomous, send representatives to regional association meetings, and they in turn elect representatives to serve on the Council of the MS Society, its ruling body. The Council meets six times a year and, together with its Executive Committee, is responsible for the smooth running of the Society and for the allocation of funds. The Council and its Executive Committee are ultimately responsible to the membership of the MS Society who can make their views known democratically through their representatives on the Council or at the Annual General Meeting.

The Chairman of the MS Society is elected at the AGM

and, with others, he or she represents the Society at national and international level, as well as being the Chairman of Council and of the Executive Committee. The Chairman is a volunteer, like all other members of the Society, but he is also a figurehead and a leader on public occasions.

The work of the Council is assisted by various specialist sub-committees. Each of these is served by experts on the subject concerned, as well as by two or three members of the Council. Another Committee deals with self-help groups and also with the affairs of younger and newly diagnosed people with MS and their families. Other committees are concerned with finance, fund raising, welfare and holiday and short stay homes.

The MS Society is advised by the Medical Research Advisory Committee, composed of research scientists and specialists in neurology. They recommend which lines of research are worth pursuing and advise the Society on media reports of 'breakthroughs', and on the many claims of treatments and cures in MS. This committee makes sure that the MS Society spends its money wisely and that it is kept up to date on all aspects of MS. It also encourages research into MS and regularly brings together scientists working in a variety of fields, so that they can share their knowledge and ideas.

The Branches at Work

However important the Council and its various committees might be, it is the branch volunteers who attempt to meet the needs of the members in their own locality, and it is they who raise much of the money that goes towards research into MS.

I have been involved in the formation of two branches in my own area, and I am kept in touch with their work through newsletters and also by attending some of the branch meetings. These two branches are quite different from one another, but both the Andover Branch and the Winchester Branch are run by a committee of volunteers. These branches have people with MS on their committees but the majority of the members have become involved because they have either relatives or friends who have MS. Each group is a mixed bunch of people who have learnt about MS through practical experience.

The Andover Branch meets regularly each month in a friendly local pub and the members enjoy a drink together, play games, and occasionally have talks and discussions on subjects which may or may not be related to MS. As well as this, the Branch publicises itself in the local press, collects money on flag days and goes in for a variety of fund-raising activities. There is a self-help group for the younger members who may wish to talk together, to share their problems and to find solutions. The Andover Branch also sponsors members who wish to attend MS workshops, and they have a specially adapted holiday caravan for the use of their members, or for other disabled people who wish to book it.

The Winchester Branch functions in a different way and reflects the needs of a different community. There is less emphasis on regular social meetings, but they raise a considerable amount of money for research each year. Both Branches have committee members who take responsibility for welfare, transport and for other activities like publicity and catering. They also have a Chairman, Secretary and Treasurer who make day-to-day administrative decisions, and who are in touch with the MS Society headquarters in London. In addition, a member of the Winchester Branch committee, who has MS herself, has been involved in a special project to advise the City of Winchester on how best to improve access and other facilities for the disabled.

At branch annual general meetings, new members of the committee are elected, ideas shared and the membership has an opportunity to make its views known, to complain or to make constructive comments for the future. Visiting speakers are invited to AGMs, and I have done my share of being one of these in other areas. No two branches are the same but, like Andover and Winchester, they all share a common purpose and a spirit of good will, despite the personality clashes and minor squabbles that are an inevitable feature of all committees!

Some branches run their own day centres, providing activities and recreations several days a week for their members, as well as a break for the relatives. Others organise fund-raising activities, sponsored events, annual dinners and a variety of entertainments, outings and other social occasions. Sometimes they can offer financial assistance to members and they may subsidise holidays or provide transport to holiday centres, some of which are run by the national MS Society.

The National Office

The staff at the National Office support the voluntary workers in the branches. They also provide up-to-date information, publicity, study days and advice on benefits, aids, holidays, diets and a whole host of other things. Staff are available at the end of the telephone and spend time counselling people who are newly diagnosed, supporting distressed relatives, or just giving advice. The National Office also organises national functions, fund-raising campaigns and appeals, and publishes a monthly Bulletin and a trendy magazine called *MS Matters*.

The Chief Executive has overall responsiblity for administration, promotion and expenditure within the agreed budget. His duties include acting as a spokesman for the Society, dealing with the media, and editing *MS Matters*. He and all his staff are at the service of the Chairman and Council of the MS Society, as well as being heavily involved in supporting the work of the branches and regional associations. They also liaise with the medical and nursing professions, with social workers and other health and social care professionals who help MS families.

Self-help Groups (formerly MS CRACK)

About twenty years ago, a young woman with MS was struck by the loneliness of young people with the disease, whom she met in hospital. She saw that they were often isolated, with no one of their own age to talk to or to compare notes with. At the same time, she was dismayed by the defeatist 'no hope' attitude that many doctors had towards MS. There seemed to be no guide-lines as to how to live with the disease in a positive manner.

This determined person was Nicole Davoude. She decided that it was essential to change attitudes both among people who had the disease and among those who were involved in helping them, such as doctors, nurses, and remedial therapists. Nicole approached the MS Society with her views and before long CRACK MS was launched, otherwise known as the Young Arm of the MS Society (and later called MS CRACK.) The idea was for the younger and newly diagnosed people to meet together in small groups and to exchange information, in order to support one another and to work actively towards changing the attitudes of society at large.

In Britain numerous self-help groups have developed from this initial idea. They are run by people who themselves have MS, together with their relatives and close friends. Groups vary greatly in how they are organised, in what they do, and also in their effectiveness.

Some groups see their main function as providing emotional support, counselling and information about MS. Others are keen to take part in fund-raising activities, in support of their branch, or in aid of special research projects. Such activities include jumble sales, craft or other sales and events like sponsored wheelchair pushes.

Some groups have a social bias, and many meet regularly in pubs or arrange a variety of outings and entertainments. Others are involved in yoga, swimming, archery, or in riding horses. In this way they encourage their members to gain in confidence, fitness, and self-respect through participating in sport. Many groups have organised publicity campaigns and distribute newsletters, posters or other advertising or educational material. There is often a good relationship with the local press who publicise the activities and needs of local groups. Sometimes a group will concentrate on building up information and knowledge about MS. Talks from visiting neurologists, social workers or occupational therapists may be arranged. Occasionally, members club together in order to obtain discounts on bulk supplies (of evening primrose oil, for instance), or even to employ their own physiotherapist or yoga instructor.

The local self-help group to which I belong has been active in the political field. We wrote a joint letter to our Member of Parliament requesting him to vote for a change in the law which would mean less discrimination against people who are disabled.

All self-help groups have in common a desire to help each person to help him- or herself and to be as independent as possible. The groups try to work closely with local branches of the MS Society and there is usually an exchange of ideas between the older, more established members in the branch, and the younger, more energetic members of the self-help group. In this way the branches themselves can remain alive and responsive to the changing needs of people with MS in their area. Several self-help groups have evolved into branches in their own right and others have provided new committee members for their branches.

Perhaps the main job of a group is to support those more recently diagnosed as having MS, who are at the beginning of their 'journey'. They can gain much from sharing their feelings and from finding out that they are not alone. Their Advisory Committee, working together with local groups, regularly runs workshops on living with MS. These explore the emotional response and the changes associated with MS, and also deal with self management and practical aids. The CRACK movement instilled a much needed sense of belonging and purpose to those of us who have MS, and helped us to feel less different from other people. It provided us all with a chance to contribute and to give to one another rather than just passively receiving as was so often the case in the past.

Other MS Charities

As well as the MS Society there are now several other charities devoted to various aspects of MS – information, newsletters, funds for specific research, special projects, local therapy centres, physiotherapy, counselling and self-help.

I have listed most of the main ones at the end of this section; many of these groups and centres are derived from a charity called ARMS (Action for Research into Multiple Sclerosis) which formed as an independent offshoot of the MS Society over twenty years ago. ARMS came into being when a number of people became dissatisfied with the MS Society at that time, and wanted to take more direct control over decisions about funding MS research. They also wanted more participation by people with MS themselves, more self-help, more emphasis on practical help and more counselling.

ARMS was largely started up by John Simpkins, whose first wife suffered from MS. It became a useful and healthy 'opposition party' to the MS Society. Like many other members of the MS Society, I also belonged to, supported and participated in ARMS except for a while when I believed that they were overemphasising the evidence that Hyperbaric Oxygen had a therapeutic role in MS.

A few years ago ARMS split into several smaller MS Therapy Centres and other groups. They often have a local bias and are fully autonomous, but still have much in common. Several of these groups continue to offer the controversial Hyperbaric Oxygen treatment, which they claim can relieve some symptoms of MS in some people.

John Simpkins now runs the MS Resource Centre (at the old ARMS address). The MSRC produces up-to-date information about MS independently from the MS Society, and a useful and thought-provoking newsletter, *Pathways*. This deals with issues ranging from cannabis to Beta Interferon and from aromatherapy to pressure sores.

The MS Society and the other MS charities jointly produced the leaflet on Beta Interferon referred to earlier in this book. However, more often they all 'do their own thing'. Perhaps a little healthy competition is good for the charities and for all of us customers. *Vive la difference!*

Other Voluntary Organisations
Besides the MS charities, many organisations provide a wide range of help for people who are sick or disabled. Details of these are available from the MS Society, from the MSRC, from hospital or Social Services departments or from Citizens' Advice Bureaux.

2 USEFUL ADDRESSES

The Multiple Sclerosis Society of Great Britain and Northern Ireland
The National Office
25 Effie Road, Fulham, London SW6 1EE. Tel: 0171-610 7171. Fax: 0171-736 9861.
UK MSS: http://www.mssociety.org.uk
UK email: Info@mssociety.org.uk

The Multiple Sclerosis Society in Scotland
2a North Charlotte Street, Edinburgh EH2 4HR. Tel: 0131-225 3600.

The Multiple Sclerosis Society Northern Ireland Office
34 Annadale Avenue, Belfast BT7 3JJ. Tel: 01232 644914.

Telephone Services
Help line: 0171-371 8000 (10am–4pm, Monday–Friday).
Counselling lines (24-hour service via referral from answer-phones listed below):
London 0171-222 3123
Midlands 0121-476 4229
Scotland 0131-226 6573

MSRC (Multiple Sclerosis Resource Centre)
4a Chapel Hill, Stanstead, Essex CM24 8AG. Tel: 01279 817101.

Other MS Charities
Association of Therapy Centres (Scotland): Tel: 01382 566283.
Federation of MS Therapy Centres: Tel. 01234 325781.
MS (Research) Charitable Trust: Tel: 01462 675613.
Northern Association of MS Therapy Centres: Tel: 0161-872 3422.
The Myelin Project: Tel: 0131-339 1316.

International Federation of Multiple Sclerosis Societies
10 Heddon Street, London W1R 7LJ. Tel: 0171-734 9120.
Fax: 0171-287 2587.
WoMS: http://www.ifmss.org.uk

RADAR (Royal Association for Disability and Rehabilitation)
12 City Forum, 250 City Road, London EC1V 8AF. Tel: 0171-250 3222.

The Disabled Living Foundation
380/384 Harrow Road, London W9 2HU. Tel: 0171-289 6111.

SPOD (Sexual and Personal Relations of People with a Disability)
286 Camden Road, London N7 1QH. Tel: 0171-607 8851/2.

Carers National Association
20–25 Glasshouse Yard, London EC1A 4JS. Tel: 0171-490 8818. Fax: 0171-490 8824.

Yoga for Health Foundation
Ickwell Bury, nr. Biggleswade, Bedfordshire SG18 9EF.
Tel: 01767 627271.

Disability Alliance Era
1st Floor East, Universal House, 89–94 Wentworth Street, London E1 7SA. Tel: 0171-247 8776. Rights advice line: 0171-247 8763.

DIAL UK (Disablement Information and Advice Line)
Park Lodge, St Catherine's Hospital, Tickhill Road, Balby, Doncaster DN4 8QN. Tel. 01302 310123.

For a full list of helpful organisations and books, apply to the MS Society.

3 FURTHER READING

ACHESON, D. (ed.) (1985). *McAlpine's Multiple Sclerosis*, third edition, Churchill Livingstone.
(This is a large and comprehensive medical reference book.)
BENZ, C. (1988). *Coping with MS*, Macdonald, Optima.
DAVOUDE, N. (1985). *Where Do I Go From Here?*, Piatkus.
DOWDIE, R., POVEY, R., AND PRETT, G. (1986). *Learning to Live with Multiple Sclerosis*, Sheldon Press.
FORSYTHE, E. (1988). *Multiple Sclerosis: Exploring Sickness and Health*, Faber & Faber.
GRAHAM, J. (1987). *Multiple Sclerosis: A Self-help Guide to its Management*, second edition, Thorsons.
KENT, H. (1985). *Yoga for the Disabled*, Thorsons.
MATHEWS, W.B. (1993). *Multiple Sclerosis: The Facts*, second edition, Oxford University Press.
MCLAUGHLIN, C. (1997). *Multiple Sclerosis — A positive approach to living with MS*, Bloomsbury.
ROBINSON, G. (1980). *Multiple Sclerosis – Simple Exercises: A Do-it-yourself Manual*, the Multiple Sclerosis Society and ARMS.
SCHAPIRO, R. (1994). *Symptom Management in Multiple Sclerosis*, second edition, Costello, Tunbridge Wells.
SCHEINBERG, L. (1983). *Multiple Sclerosis: A Guide for Patients and their Families*, Raven Press, New York, USA.

SHERIDAN, P. (ed.) (1995). *Multiple Sclerosis: Research in Progress, 1993–1994*, IFMSS.

SIBLEY, W.A. (1994). *Therapeutic Claims in Multiple Sclerosis*, third edition, Demos Publications, New York, USA.

SIMONS, A. (ed.) (1984). *Multiple Sclerosis: Psychological and Social Aspects*, Heinemann Medical Books.

STEWART, W. (1985). *Counselling in Rehabilitation*, Croom Helm.

JOURNALS

MS Management, twice a year. Published by IFMSS.

MS Matters, quarterly. Published by the MS Society.

Pathways, quarterly. Published by MSRC.

Update, twice a year. Published by IFMSS.

Index

(Page numbers in bold indicate an illustration)